W9-CBA-887

Peripheral Vascular Surgery

Atlas of Operative Surgery Series

Series Editor
R. Scott Jones, M.D.
Professor and Chairman
Department of Surgery
University of Virginia School of Medicine
Charlottesville, Virginia

Several other titles under development.

Peripheral Vascular Surgery

Wade C. Lamberth, Jr., M.D.

Donald B. Doty, M.D.

Illustrated by
Christy Krames, M.A.

YEAR BOOK MEDICAL PUBLISHERS, INC.
Chicago • London • Boca Raton

Copyright © 1987 by Year Book Medical Publishers, Inc. All rights reserved. No part of this publication may be reproduced, stored in a retrieval system, or transmitted, in any form or by any means—electronic, mechanical, photocopying, recording, or otherwise—without prior written permission from the publisher. Printed in the United States of America.

1 2 3 4 5 6 7 8 9 0 Y C 91 90 89 88 87

Library of Congress Cataloging-in-Publication Data

Lamberth, Wade C., Jr.
    Peripheral vascular surgery.

    Includes bibliographies and index.
    1. Blood-vessels—Surgery. I. Doty, Donald B.
II. Title. [DNLM: 1. Vascular Surgery—atlases.
WG 17 L222p]
RD598.5.L35 1987   617'.413   86-33947
ISBN 0-8151-5324-4

Sponsoring Editor: Daniel J. Doody
Manager, Copyediting Services: Frances M. Perveiler
Copyeditor: Francis A. Byrne
Production Manager, Text and Reference/Periodicals: Etta Worthington
Proofroom Supervisor: Shirley E. Taylor

About the Authors

Wade C. Lamberth, Jr., M.D.

Wade C. Lamberth, Jr., received his M.D. from the University of Alabama Medical School in 1968, and subsequently completed his internship and residency in surgery at the University of Alabama Medical Center in Birmingham. Dr. Lamberth completed fellowships in peripheral vascular surgery and thoracic surgery at the University of Iowa Hospitals where he was then appointed Assistant Professor of Surgery, Division of Thoracic and Cardiovascular Surgery. Currently, he is Attending Surgeon at Flowers Hospital and Southeast Alabama Medical Center, Dothan, Alabama

Donald B. Doty, M.D.

Donald B. Doty received his M.D. from Stanford University College of Medicine in 1962, and completed his internship and residency in surgery at the University of Southern California—Los Angeles County Medical Center. Dr. Doty completed a fellowship in thoracic surgery at the University of Alabama Medical Center in Birmingham. Thereafter he assumed a position of Professor of Surgery, Division of Thoracic and Cardiovascular Surgery, University of Iowa Hospitals. He is currently Clinical Professor of Surgery, Division of Thoracic and Cardiovascular Surgery, University of Utah School of Medicine, and is Chairman, Division of Thoracic and Cardiovascular Surgery, LDS Hospital, Salt Lake City, Utah.

About the Illustrator

Christy Krames, M.A.

Christy Krames received a Master of Arts in Medical Illustration from the University of Texas Health Sciences Center at Dallas in 1981. She was the Staff Medical Illustrator, Department of Surgery, University of Iowa Hospitals and is currently a freelance medical illustrator in Salt Lake City, Utah.

To our teacher of the art of surgery,
John W. Kirklin, M.D.,
who taught and exemplified excellence in operative technique,
and to our patients,
who have shown us how the conduct of the operation
determines the postoperative course.

Series Introduction

Many practicing surgeons and surgical teachers will remember the *Handbooks of Operative Surgery* originally published in the early 1950s. This series of books written by respected clinical surgeons represented multiple disciplines of surgery. The objective of the original Handbook series was to describe the essentials of pre- and postoperative care and to provide lucid illustrations of operative techniques. Each author included careful descriptions of his operative techniques and analysis of indications for surgery, and discussed the common problems associated with the disease and its treatment. The *Handbook of Operative Surgery* provided surgical residents an excellent day-to-day reference for preparation for operating room assignments. In addition, busy practitioners found the format and content of the *Handbook* convenient, practical, and easy to use for reference and review.

One of my teachers, Dr. Julian Johnson, and his associate, Dr. Charles Kirby, wrote the volume in the series entitled *Surgery of the Chest*. My fellow residents and I made this book our constant companion.

Since the 1950s and 1960s when most of the *Handbooks of Operative Surgery* were written and revised, the practice of surgery has changed drastically. Some operations of that era are now obsolete, while new approaches developed in every field. In addition to surgical techniques, devices to support intraoperative management, diagnostic imaging, and pre- and postoperative care have all undergone remarkable changes and progress during the preceding one and a half decades. Because of the extraordinary utility and educational success of the original *Handbook of Operative Surgery* series, and the extent of changes in surgery since that time, Year Book Medical Publishers is undertaking a complete reorganization and revision of the Handbook series to feature new authors and completely new and updated material, presented in a more contemporary format. The components of this new *Atlas of Operative Surgery* series will be intended primarily for general surgery residents and general surgeons, and the new editions will pay particular attention to intraoperative management of diseases encountered by practicing general surgeons.

The Lamberth and Doty volume on peripheral vascular surgery provides an outstanding initiation of this major new effort. It clearly reflects the mission and intent of the revitalized *Atlas of Operative Surgery* series with detailed descriptions of all of the vascular operations likely to be performed by general surgeons and most vascular surgery specialists. The lucid clarity of the outstanding artwork accompanied by the complete and thoughtful narration of these leading vascular surgeons provide a major contribution to the field. This complete and authoritative volume will greatly assist residents in preparing for current-day operating room assignments and help surgeons provide their patients the best care possible.

R. Scott Jones, M.D.
Professor and Chairman
Department of Surgery
University of Virginia School
   of Medicine
Charlottesville, Virginia

Preface

This book is an atlas of operations performed on the vascular system. The purpose of the text and illustrations is to provide information that will allow the novice surgeon to enter unfamiliar peripheral vascular operations more confidently, and to provide material that the experienced surgeon may review prior to infrequently performed procedures. The operations are presented in detailed step-by-step fashion as clearly and concisely as possible. The techniques described are methods that we have found to be reliable and reproducible. We have attempted to include all operations of proven value and practiced by established vascular surgeons. Unproven, experimental, or personally unique operations are not included. The procedures described should be representative of safe and effective methods for performing the scope of operations included in vascular surgery.

The format for the presentation of the material is consistent throughout. Each chapter is introduced by title and graphics that define the area of the vascular system to be detailed. The steps of the operations are presented as they would be performed in text, which could resemble a report of operation. The text is also the legend for illustrations of the operation that are displayed on the facing page. The important features of surgical anatomy and the pathology to be treated introduce the set of illustrations. The drawings are in the anatomic perspective as though the patient's head were at the top of the page. Cross-sectional anatomy is illustrated from the perspective of looking up from the feet similar to the convention used in axial tomography.

Since we decided upon an atlas format, information regarding diagnosis, pathophysiology, pre- and postoperative care, indications for operation, and results are not included. Likewise, references are not included. The presentations of the operations are as we perform them, and represent a synthesis of techniques devised by many innovative surgeons. The emphasis is upon how to perform operations with hope and expectation that this information will provide a ready reference for the vascular surgeon.

WADE C. LAMBERTH, JR., M.D.
DONALD B. DOTY, M.D.

Contents

Vascular Techniques

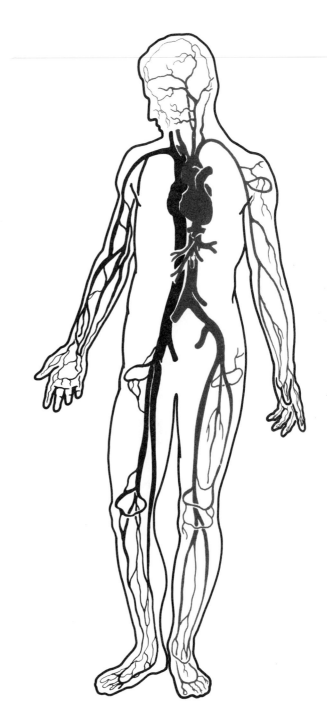

General Principles

Fig 1–1. Operations on the blood vessels demand consistent precise operative technique. Since many of the operations will be performed on vessels damaged by atherosclerotic change in the arterial wall or on naturally thin walled veins, the tissue is difficult to handle and precise technique must be used. A surgeon soon learns that precision and accuracy in performing the procedure in the operating room has a great effect on the situations encountered after the procedure is over. The events in the operating room generally determine the course afterwards. Thus, it is incumbent upon all who operate on the circulatory system to have carefully organized treatment plans for the various pathologic conditions that are predicated upon reproducible operations. The operation should be planned well in advance and based upon the surgeon's prior experience as to what usually works for him. Options should be considered depending upon the conditions encountered, but as a general rule, it is best to make the situations conform to the plan of operation rather than "making it up" as the operation proceeds.

Operations on the circulatory system often consist of many steps and maneuvers causing them to be lengthy because of the many things that have to be done. The complexity of the operation is usually related to the complexity of the disease process that is being treated. There is a tendency to allow these operations to become tedious in situations where the disease is extensive and the blood vessels are small. The experienced and efficient vascular surgeon does not become distracted by the disease or the operative situation and finds means to make difficult things appear easy. This is done by having a clear treatment plan which has been shown by previous experience to be reproducible, not allowing the pathology encountered to deviate the plan or to bog down the operation, making every maneuver or step lead to logical progression of the operation, not creating problems by foolish technical blunders, and by striving for accuracy rather than unobtainable perfection.

Perfect visualization of the morphology in the operative field is essential to achieving accuracy in operative repair. The surgeon must assure that his own vision has proper acuity. Vision is remarkably enhanced by optical magnification through the use of 2.5 to 3.5 × operating loupes. The small field of vision in these magnifying devices tends to focus attention to the critical area of the operating field. Peripheral vision is obviously sacrificed using operating loupes so that their use may best be restricted to points in the operation when accurate dissection or suture control is desired. Intense, focused light is supplied to the critical area of the operating field by the use of fiberoptic headlamps adjusted to illuminate the field of vision of the operating loupes or the most comfortable working field when the loupes are not in use. Deep or unusual exposures may be flooded with light which would otherwise be shrouded or hidden from overhead illumination. Good vision into a well lighted area combined with proper "setting up" of the operating field by appropriate tissue retraction allows the operation to proceed and without distraction.

The use of heparin administered intravenously to achieve systemic anticoagulant effect is favored for nearly all operations on blood vessels. The dose of heparin is based on experience that 100 to 200 units/kg will achieve anticoagulant effect that will prevent coagulation of blood during the period required for completion of most procedures requiring vascular occlusion. For critical procedures, especially on small arteries or veins, a dose of heparin on the high side (150 to 200 units/kg) is used and the anticoagulant effect is monitored by activated clotting time of whole blood. Activated clotting time in excess of 400 seconds will prevent blood clotting and the consumption of clotting factors. Activated clotting times in the range of 200 seconds are probably adequate for less critical operating situations.

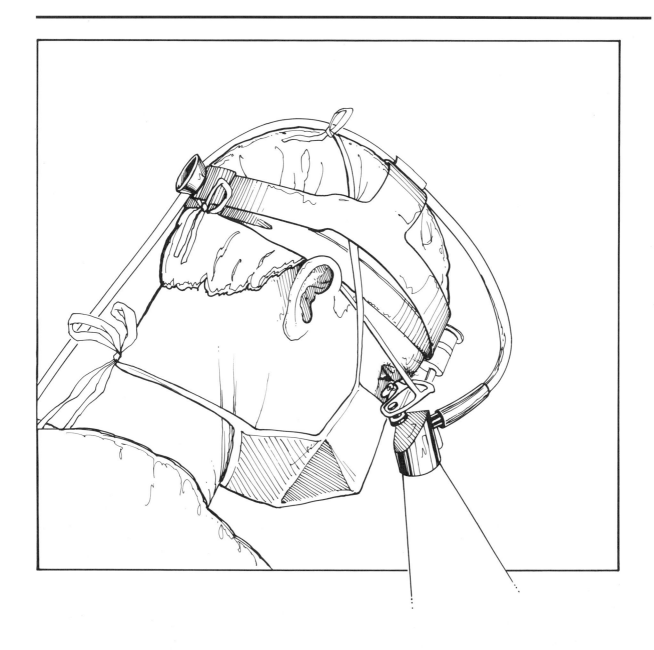

Instruments

Fig 1–2. The peripheral vascular tray usually displays an array of instruments designed for a multitude of unique situations encountered in operations on the vascular system. There is an immense variety of sizes and shapes of vascular instruments, yet the surgeon soon finds that he uses only a few familiar and trusted devices for most operations.

A. One of the most versatile atraumatic vascular clamps employed is the DeBakey curved aneurysm clamp. The 10½-inch model is just about right for most circumstances. The clamp can be used to occlude the aorta with minimal dissection alongside the vessel. In the emergency situation or where there is dense inflammatory tissue around the aorta, this clamp is most helpful. It occludes the aorta by bringing in the sides of the vessel. This provides a vertical orientation of the open end of the vessel that can be somewhat awkward for vascular reconstruction. Disease in the infrarenal abdominal aorta tends to deviate the aorta away from the anterior aspect of the spine just below the renal arteries so that control of the aorta from the side is easily achieved. Several so-called sidewinder clamps have been designed for this purpose. Dissection of the posterior surface of the aorta is required, but the occlusion may then be applied in an anterior-posterior fashion providing a better orientation of the open end of the aorta for reconstruction.

B. Possibly the most versatile and frequently used vascular clamp is the DeBakey 7-inch straight jaw 35-degree angled peripheral vascular clamp. Four of these clamps should be in every vascular instrument tray. These clamps may be used to occlude just about any blood vessel in the body from the aorta to the carotid or popliteal artery. Occlusion of deep, vertically oriented arteries such as the internal iliac or profunda femoris arteries is nicely accomplished with a modified Henley clamp.

C. Partial occluding clamps are also available in a variety of sizes and shapes. These clamps may be used to isolate a portion of a large blood vessel for vascular reconstruction, to totally occlude smaller vessels to eliminate a second clamp in a small operating field, or to pass around blood vessels while achieving vascular control. At least four sizes are required: extra large (Glover appendage clamp), large (Lambert-Kay aortic anastomosis clamp), medium (Derra anastomosis clamp), and small (Cooley pediatric anastomosis clamp).

D. The proper use of vascular clamps will assure their "atraumatic" function. Atherosclerotic disease tends to be eccentric. Generally, the atherosclerotic plaque is worse on the posterior wall of the artery. It is most correct to apply the clamp in an orientation that will compress the soft, less diseased wall against the atherosclerotic plaque. It is incorrect to compress the vessel alongside of the plaque. Vascular clamps are usually constructed with a double row of low serrations that cause minimal tissue crush when jaws of the clamps are closed onto a blood vessel. Multiple grooves in the closure mechanism of these clamps provide a means for graded closure and opening. The clamp should only be closed to a point sufficient to occlude the blood vessel so as to avoid tissue trauma or the possibility of fracture of an atherosclerotic plaque. Similarly, opening of the clamp can be gradual with partial reperfusion to avoid the consequences of arterial hypotension with sudden reflow to a vascular bed.

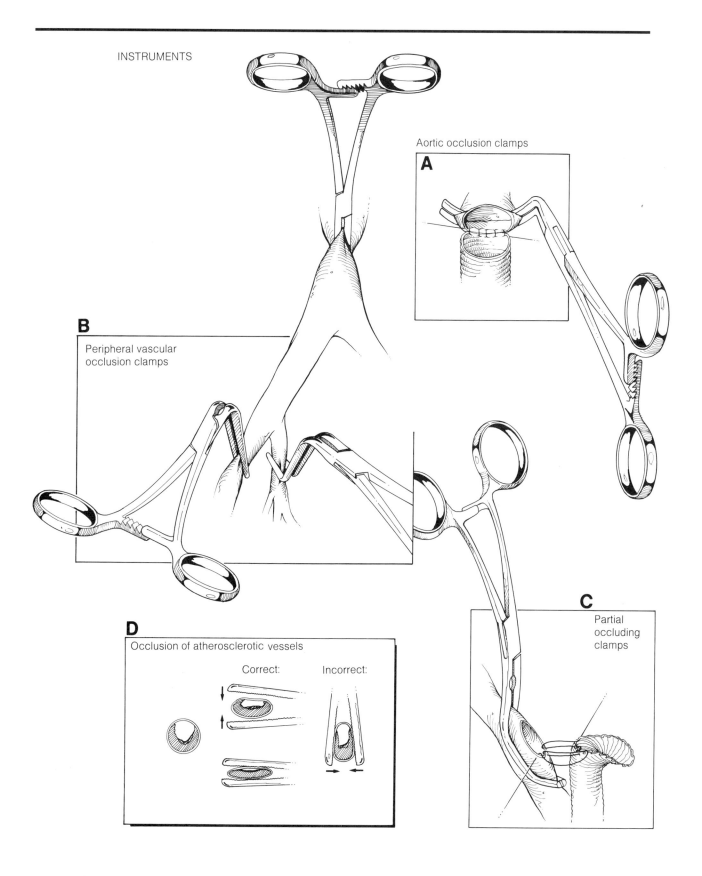

Aortic occlusion clamps

A

B

Peripheral vascular
occlusion clamps

C

Partial
occluding
clamps

D

Occlusion of atherosclerotic vessels

Correct: Incorrect:

Fig 1–2, E. Occlusion of vascular prostheses is a special problem because the tiny teeth of atraumatic vascular clamps tend to perforate the film of thrombus which seals up the interstices of these grafts. The soft jaw clamps (Fogarty) are best for this purpose. The rubber inserts for the clamp occlude the prosthesis without perforation. The fabric of the prosthesis is rough enough to prevent slippage of the clamp.

F. Occlusion of small vessels requires a small device that has gentle tension in the jaws so as not to damage the intima of the small artery or vein. The Diethrich micro-coronary bulldog clamp is a most valuable device for this application. This clamp is often used with only enough mobilization alongside the blood vessel to allow closure of the clamp. It is often used in combination with the Cooley pediatric anastomosis clamp.

G. Endarterectomy requires a spatula that can be used to separate the atheromatous plaque from the adventitial layer of the artery with neither fragmentation of the plaque nor perforation of the adventitia. Several instruments have been designed specifically for the purpose, but most of them are either too small and narrow or unnecessarily complicated and varied to be uniformly practical. For most large arteries, the Freer septum elevator (otolaryngological), double-ended, sharp variety is most satisfactory. The spatula shaped ends are appropriately rounded yet with enough sharpness of the edge to cut away the plaque with ease. For tiny vessels, the Wheeler cyclodialysis spatula (ophthalmological) is useful because of its size and malleability.

H. Accurate performance of vascular anastomosis where small suture loops must be placed into small blood vessels that may also have difficult to manage tissue in the wall is enhanced by the use of a positive release needle driver. The Castroviejo type needle driver with smooth diamond inserts in the jaws is best. The jaws should be fine but not so delicate as to provide enough gripping area to hold the needle during passage through sclerotic or calcareous tissue. Smooth jaws are preferred so that the thin metal of the needle on fine suture is not damaged by closure of the needle driver. Short (5½-inch) needle drivers are used almost exclusively, but medium length (7-inch) devices are also available.

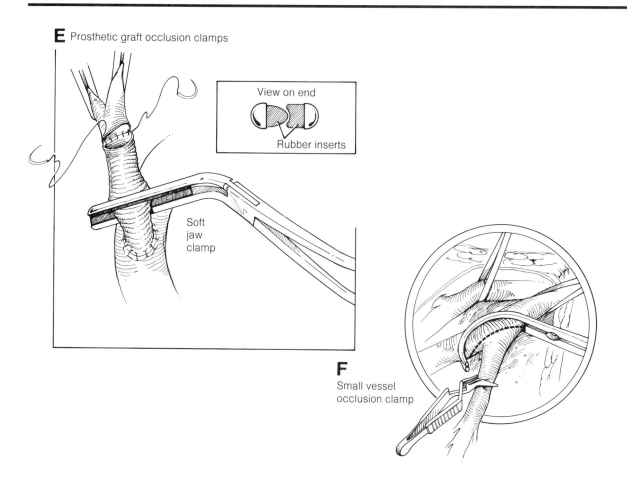

E Prosthetic graft occlusion clamps

View on end

Rubber inserts

Soft
jaw
clamp

F
Small vessel
occlusion clamp

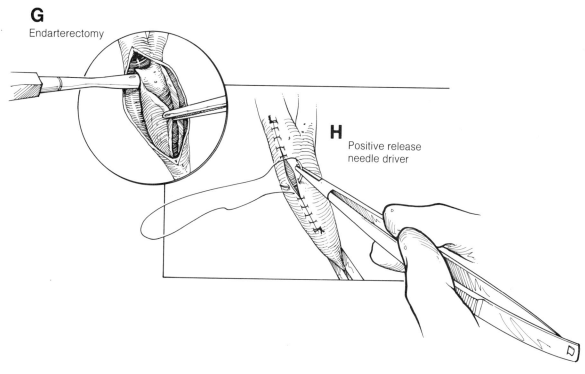

G
Endarterectomy

H Positive release
needle driver

Exposure and Control of Blood Vessels

Fig 1–3. Techniques of tissue dissection to gain exposure and control of blood vessels are critical to safe and accurate operations in vascular surgery. Basic principles of thorough visualization of the operative field and clean separation of tissue planes must be diligently applied. Compromise of the exposure and division of tissue without visualization usually creates problems which on certain occasions ruins the operation. The operator must demand of himself consistent, complete exposure of the area of dissection and use his assistants and self-retaining retraction devices in thoughtful ways in order to achieve that required exposure.

A. The principle of traction and counter traction on tissue to expose the dissection plane is always applied and very useful around blood vessels. Both arteries and veins are fixed into tissue planes by connective tissue which courses perpendicular from the blood vessel walls to the surrounding tissue structures. The basic technique of blood vessel dissection then requires exposure of these transverse connecting fibers. Atraumatic vascular forceps (DeBakey) are used to grip the vessel on the adventitial surface only and pull it to the side to expose the transverse connecting fibers. These transverse fibers are often referred to as the ''begging'' fibers as in begging to be cut. The fibers are divided by scissors (Lilly dissecting scissors). Sharp dissection is used nearly uniformly. Blunt techniques are used sparingly to separate tissue planes. When used, the scissors are opened perpendicular to the blood vessel to expose any perpendicularly oriented branches as the tissues separate, rather than opening the scissors longitudinal to the vessel which will tear off branches prior to their identification.

B. Large vessels such as the aorta are better retracted using fingers on gauze sponge technique. This provides traction against the vessel distributed over a wider area with minimal trauma to the vessel wall.

C. Once a vessel is mobilized sufficiently to encircle it, a vessel loop (silicone strip or Dacron fabric tape) can be passed around and used for retraction. Exposure may be enhanced by having two loops retracted to expose the tissue between them.

Methods of Arteriotomy

A. The safest method of performing arteriotomy is by incision with scalpel. A #15 scalpel blade is used to sequentially incise the layers of the vessel wall. The blade must be new and sharp so that it accurately cuts through the tissue. Excessive pressure against the vessel or a blunted blade may allow it to abruptly enter the lumen which may cause injury to the back wall. Entry of the lumen is confirmed by escape of blood.

B. The arteriotomy is extended to appropriate length using Potts vascular scissors. A variety of scissor tip angles are available so that the arteriotomy can be extended without awkwardness. The scissors should be inserted to the exact length of desired incision and the cut made to the tip of the scissors so that it is full thickness and clean at the apex of the arteriotomy.

C. Stab incision for arteriotomy is often performed for convenience and simplicity. It is best used in larger vessels. The hazards of this technique include injury of the back wall of the vessel and failure to accurately enter the lumen of an atherosclerotic vessel with disruption of an atherosclerotic plaque rather than actually opening up the arteriotomy to the blood flow pathway.

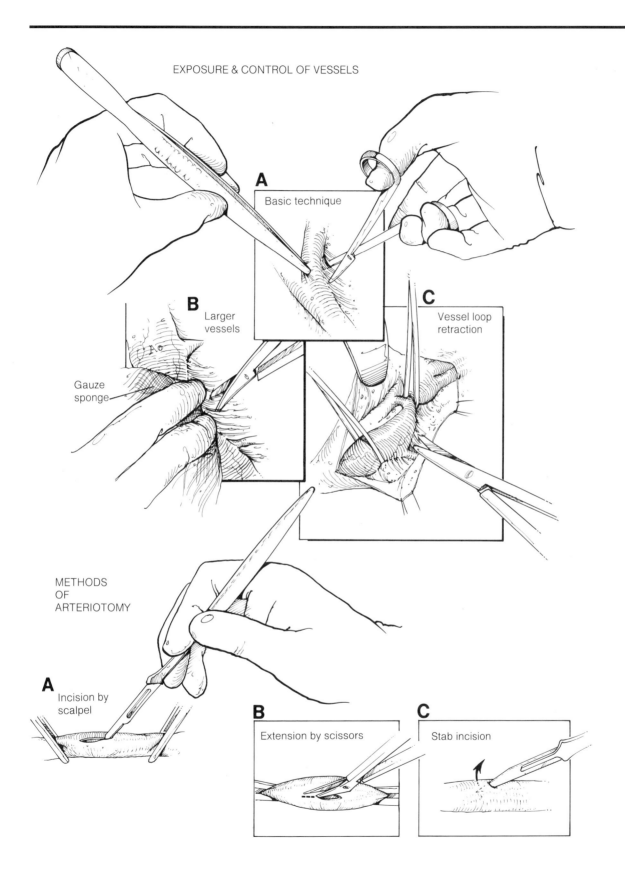

A Basic technique

B Larger vessels

Gauze sponge

C Vessel loop retraction

METHODS OF ARTERIOTOMY

A Incision by scalpel

B Extension by scissors

C Stab incision

Technique of Anastomosis

Fig 1–4. Vascular reconstruction almost always involves techniques that join tubular structures in anastomosis. It is imperative that reproducible techniques of anastomosis be established and followed with some persistence. Continuous suture techniques using monofilament suture material are favored almost exclusively except in some small vessels where interrupted suture technique can be adapted appropriately. Simple over and over suture technique is employed so that the edges of tissue or graft approximate accurately. Everting techniques using mattress sutures are avoided. As a general principle, the needle is passed through the intimal surface of the host vessel to the outside so that the intima will be pressed against the media rather than lifted away. Certain circumstances of exposure and access will dictate that following this inside-out principle will be awkward and could place unnecessary torque against the curve of the needle and with the possibility of creating trauma to the intimal surface as it passes through the vessel wall. These circumstances will suggest that the real principles that should be followed are to prevent injury to the intimal surface and to avoid atheromatous plaque disruption by passing the needle through the vessel wall accurately while following the curve of the needle with the least possible awkwardness. Sometimes it will be necessary to use an outside-in technique to follow these principles. This is most safe when the arterial wall is near normal with minimal atheromatous plaque.

A. *End-to-side anastomosis, beveled.* The most commonly performed anastomosis is the joining of a beveled graft to a longitudinal arteriotomy. A standard technique is used employing placement of the initial five suture loops between the "heel" of the graft and the end of the opening in the vessel. Two stitches are placed to the side opposite the operator, the third precisely through the apex of the incision parallel to the vessel, and the fourth and fifth stitches on the side toward the operator. The graft is held apart from the vessel during placement of these suture loops to provide exposure of the apex of the arteriotomy.

B. Pulling up of the suture loops accurately approximates graft to vessel. Lateral traction on the free ends of the suture pulls apart the edges of the vessel incision and enhances exposure of the rest of the anastomosis.

C. Completion of anastomosis involves accurate placement of approximately five suture loops around the "toe" of the graft. The suture loops may be left slightly loose so that the intimal surface and the edge of the graft may be accurately visualized with placement of each stitch. The suturing should proceed like spokes on a cart wheel around the apex of the anastomosis. Suturing should proceed in an orderly progression for accurate approximation of the structures. There is no advantage of many extra stitches which makes the procedure tedious and adds unnecessary foreign material (suture) to the anastomosis and multiplies the possibility of tissue trauma. Completion of the anastomosis by joining the suture ends by knot should be accurate and tight enough to approximate the tissues without narrowing the anastomosis.

D. *End-to-end anastomosis.* End-to-end anastomosis of large vessels or graft is performed by simple continuous suture technique. The back row of the anastomosis is completed by placing all the suture loops prior to approximating the ends of the vessels. Typically, the stitches are placed from the outside-in on the graft so that the needle may pass through the intimal surface of the host vessel. When joining two vessels with normal vessel wall morphology, it may be easier to sew from the inside of the vessel below or to the operator's right. (*Continued on page 12.*)

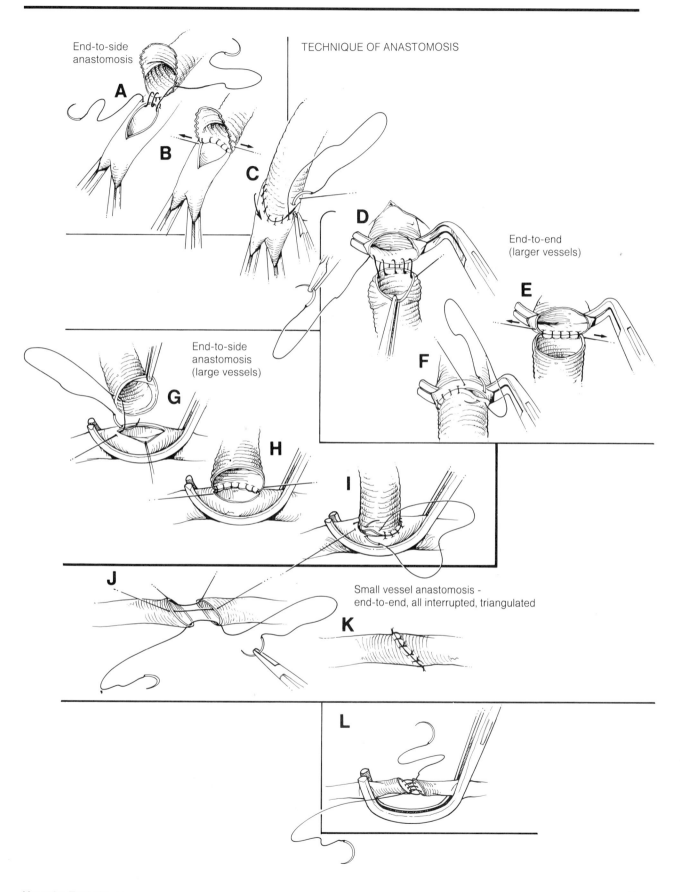

End-to-side
anastomosis

A

B

C

TECHNIQUE OF ANASTOMOSIS

D

End-to-end
(larger vessels)

E

F

End-to-side
anastomosis
(large vessels)

G

H

I

J

K

Small vessel anastomosis -
end-to-end, all interrupted, triangulated

L

E. The vessels are approximated by pulling up the suture loops of the back wall. Suture loop tension may be adjusted with a nerve hook. The accuracy of tissue approximation will be evident at this point.

F. The anterior row of sutures are placed in the most convenient fashion to complete the anastomosis.

G. *End-to-side anastomosis, nonbeveled.* Joining tubular structures in end-to-side is most simply accomplished by sewing from the inside on the back row of the anastomosis. Setting up the anastomosis on the initial three needle passes makes the difference between ease and difficulty. The needles at each end of the suture are passed from the inside-out at the apex of the longitudinal incision and the side of the vessel or graft to be joined. The needle on the graft side is then brought back into the longitudinal incision from outside-in. Sometimes a retraction suture placed in the middle of the longitudinal incision on the side toward the operator sets up the exposure.

H. The back row of the anastomosis is constructed by passing the needle from the inside surface of the end vessel through to the inside of the longitudinal incision.

I. The anterior row of the anastomosis is completed in the most convenient fashion, removing the retraction stitch at the point it is crossed during the suturing.

J. *Small vessel anastamoses.* End-to-end anastomosis of small vessels is traditionally accomplished by triangulation technique and all interrupted sutures. The vessel circumferences are divided into approximate thirds by fine suture passed between the vessels.

K. The spaces between the triangulation stitches are filled in with interrupted sutures.

L. Continuous suture technique can also be effectively employed. Holding both vessels in a single vascular clamp makes the anastomosis easier.

Carotid Endarterectomy

2

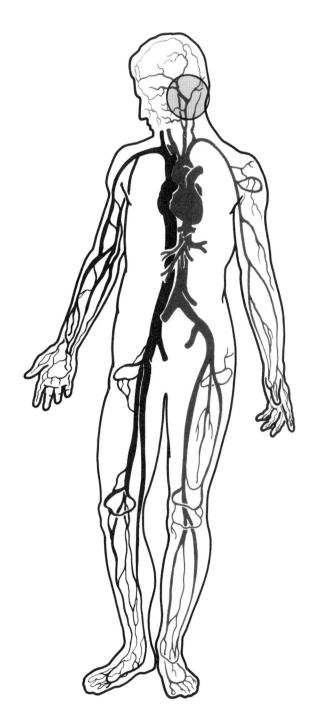

Fig 2–1. Atherosclerotic plaques producing stenosis of the carotid artery and ulceration of the intima causing cerebral or ocular embolism are treated by endarterectomy. An incision paralleling the anterior margin of the sternocleidomastoid muscle affords maximum exposure of the entire cervical course of the carotid artery. A cosmetic skin line (transverse) incision made toward the upper edge of the larynx may be used.

A. The anterior edge of the sternocleidomastoid muscle is completely mobilized. The facial vein is divided and the internal jugular vein mobilized laterally. The ansa cervicalis (hypoglossi) lies over the carotid artery and is a good guide to the hypoglossal nerve which crosses the internal and external carotid arteries in a transverse direction. Branches of the external carotid artery are controlled with loop suture.

B. The common carotid artery is controlled with a vessel loop. The internal and external branches of the carotid artery are controlled beyond the palpable extent of atheromatous disease and encircled with the vessel loop. Dissection should avoid tissues between the carotid branches to preserve the carotid body mechanism and its nerve. The surfaces of the carotid artery are exposed by retraction of tissues away from the artery with forceps and division of transverse connecting fibers with scissors. Blunt dissection is avoided. The artery should not be elevated from its bed. The carotid bifurcation is minimally manipulated to prevent atheroembolism.

C. Heparin is administered. Angled peripheral vascular clamps (DeBakey) are applied to the common and external carotid arteries. Back perfusion pressure in the internal carotid artery is measured by needle puncture. An infant anastomosis clamp (Cooley) is placed on the internal carotid artery. The arteriotomy is made laterally on the common carotid artery. The arteriotomy is extended to the internal carotid artery beyond the atheromatous plaque with Potts scissors.

C′. Use of a shunt is controversial. We have employed a shunt when continuously monitored electroencephalogram shows diminution or slowing of electrical signals from any portion of the brain. Tourniquets are placed on the vessel loops. The shunt catheter is placed into the internal carotid artery, then into the common carotid artery. The catheter is advanced carefully into the internal carotid artery lest a flap be created in the intima.

D. The atheromatous plaque is separated from the carotid artery by dissection in the layer between media and adventitia. A Freer septum elevator is the most useful instrument. Optical magnification (2.5 to 3.5 ×) provides accurate visualization. Forceps are used to retract the vessel wall as the plaque is pushed away. The dissection is started in the common carotid artery. The plaque is completely encircled. The plaque is divided at the lowest extent to the arteriotomy. Scissors are used to cut the plaque at the point of separation leaving a smooth, well attached proximal edge in the common carotid artery.

E. The plaque is separated from the external carotid artery to a tapered end point.

F. Separation of the plaque from the internal carotid artery is the most critical maneuver. As the end of the plaque is approached, a transition is made to a more superficial layer in the intima-media so that the plaque will come away and leave a firm attachment of the intima layer. The transition must be consciously made rather than leaving separation to chance. The Freer elevator or scissors are used to cut into the edge of the plaque at one side of the arteriotomy at a more superficial layer. The plaque can then be thinned or "feathered" out to a clean separation with the underlying intima tightly attached. Attention to this detail will avoid the necessity of "tacking down" the intima.

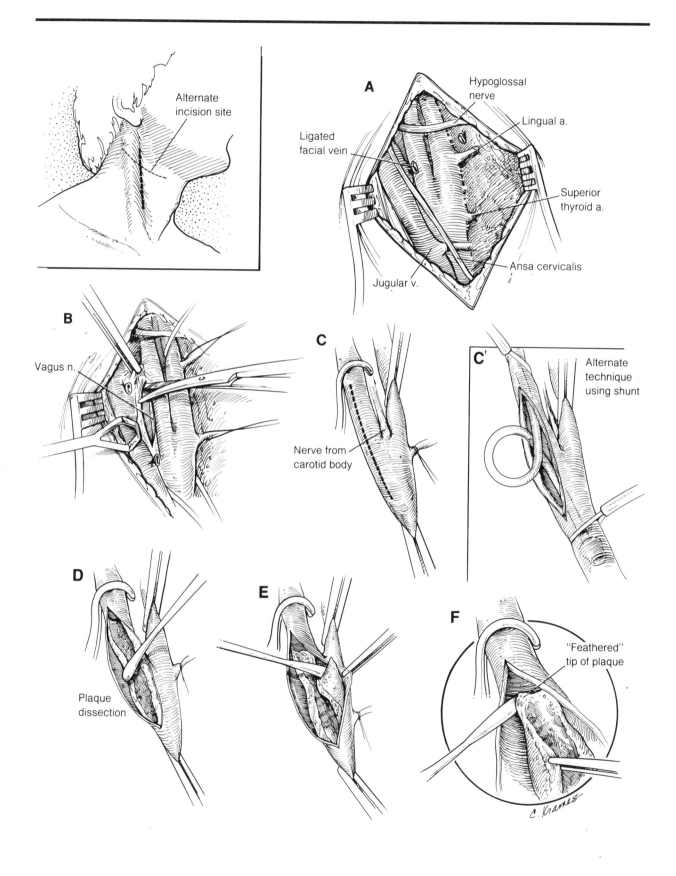

Alternate incision site

A

Hypoglossal nerve

Lingual a.

Ligated facial vein

Superior thyroid a.

Ansa cervicalis

Jugular v.

B

Vagus n.

C

Nerve from carotid body

C'

Alternate technique using shunt

D

Plaque dissection

E

F

"Feathered" tip of plaque

C. Krames

Fig 2–1, G. Fragments of transverse smooth muscle fibers of the media are left attached to the wall of the artery during the most meticulous dissection of the plaque. These bits of loose debris are pulled away from the artery with forceps. A Kuettner dissector may also be used to gently dislodge these fibers. The point of proximal transection of the plaque is examined along with the distal endpoints. Flooding the artery with saline irrigation will expose any remaining loose fragments.

H. The arteriotomy is closed by continuous stitch of 6/0 polypropylene. Needles at each end of the suture are passed from the inside of the artery at the distal end and secured by knot. The initial stitches in the internal carotid artery must be carefully placed using the smallest possible amount of the vessel wall consistent with security of the arteriotomy closure to obtain maximum vessel diameter. Once into the carotid bifurcation and below, more substantial stitches into the vessel wall may be taken. Prior to final closure of the arteriotomy, the occlusion clamps are removed to back bleed any debris out the arteriotomy. The clamps are opened sequentially with the internal carotid artery last to be perfused. The flow dynamics of the completed repair are evaluated by Doppler ultrasound. The ultrasound crystal is placed directly on the carotid artery and its branches to evaluate both systolic and diastolic flow velocity.

I. It is sometimes necessary to use a vein patch to close the arteriotomy when direct suture of the internal carotid artery would result in a stenotic lumen.

J. Excessive length of the internal carotid artery, which results in kinking, may be associated with atheromatous changes of the carotid artery. After endarterectomy performed in the usual technique, the excessive length of the internal carotid artery may be removed and an anastomosis created in end-to-end fashion to the carotid bulb. Sometimes the removal of the plaque will result in redundant internal carotid artery with inadequate flow dynamics. This may also be treated by resection and anastomosis.

K. Recurrence of carotid artery stenosis occasionally occurs. Reoperation for the relief of stenosis is best accomplished by patch angioplasty. The previous arteriotomy is reopened, allowing the stenotic area to separate. The arteriotomy is closed by vein patch angioplasty using a small piece of the saphenous vein.

L. Patch angioplasty employing polytetrafluoroethylene graft is also an acceptable alternative. The patch is attached to the arteriotomy by placing the initial five stitches around the distal end of the arteriotomy with the patch held away from the vessel for maximum accuracy of suture placement. The patch is approximated to the vessel by tightening the suture loops. Suture material is 6/0 or 5/0 polypropylene depending on the thickness of the vessel wall. The remainder of the arteriotomy is completed in usual fashion.

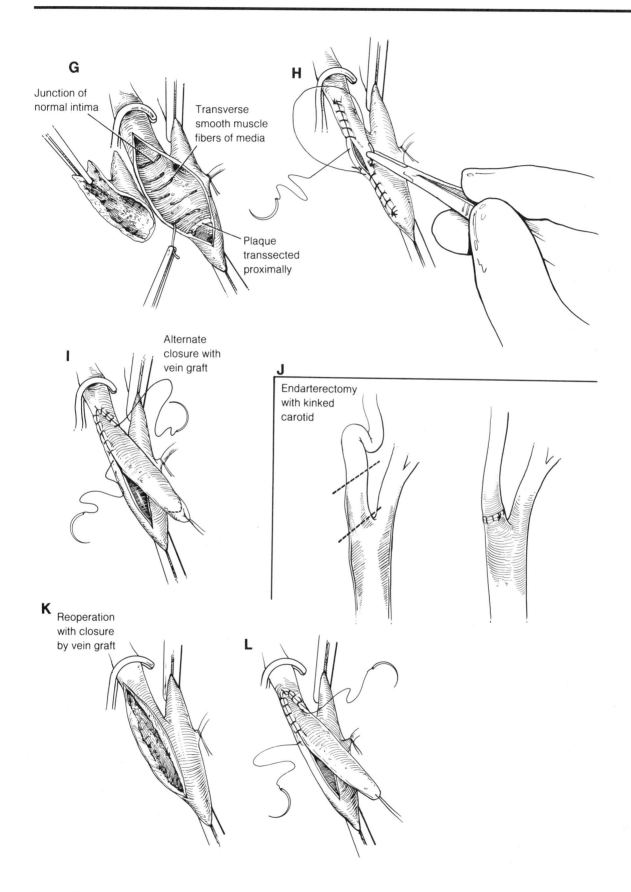

G

Junction of normal intima

Transverse smooth muscle fibers of media

Plaque transsected proximally

H

I

Alternate closure with vein graft

J

Endarterectomy with kinked carotid

K Reoperation with closure by vein graft

L

External Carotid Endarterectomy

3

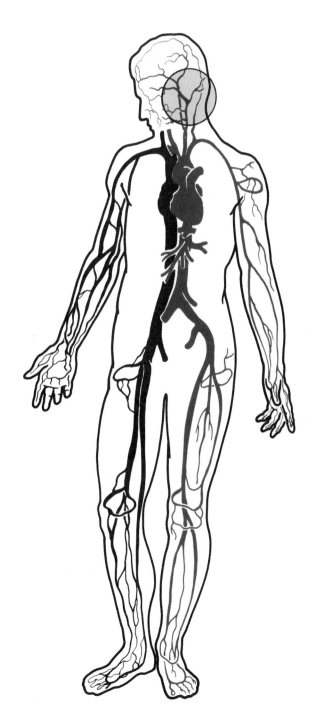

Fig 3–1. The external carotid artery is approached through an incision paralleling the anterior border of the sternocleidomastoid muscle. This provides optimal exposure of the length of the common carotid artery and the internal and external branches of the artery. Alternatively, a more cosmetic skin line incision may be used.

A. Cerebral or ocular symptoms related to stenosis of the external carotid artery may occur when there is occlusion of the internal carotid artery and major cerebral blood supply is via the external carotid artery through collateral circulation, especially through the ocular orbit. Thrombosis of the internal carotid artery may result in retention of a small cul de sac which may accumulate platelet-fibrin debris which can embolize through the external carotid artery. All the major branches of the external carotid artery may be controlled by dissection along the course of the artery. Arteriotomy begins on the common carotid artery and is extended to the external carotid artery beyond the atheromatous disease.

B. Branches of the external carotid artery are occluded with loop suture ligature. A Diethrich vascular clamp is used on the external carotid artery. A DeBakey 35-degree angle peripheral vascular clamp is used to occlude the common carotid artery, and no clamp is required for the internal carotid artery. Endarterectomy is started in the common carotid artery. Optical magnification may be used to visualize the dissection plane accurately. The plaque is divided proximally, leaving a clean and undisturbed attachment of the unresected plaque to the carotid artery. The plaque is mobilized away from the vessel wall by dissection in the media-adventitia layer with a Freer septum elevator. The dissection is taken into the internal carotid artery for a short distance.

C. The plaque is broken off from the internal carotid artery. The critical part of dissection of the plaque is the separation of the distal endpoint from the external carotid artery. The plaque is "feathered" by taking the dissection more superficially into the intima-media layer. The plaque may be removed from a tightly adherent intima distally.

D. The internal carotid artery is separated from the common carotid artery by dividing the artery at its origin.

E. The origin of the internal carotid artery is closed by continuous suture using 6/0 polypropylene. This maneuver is designed to eliminate the potential cul de sac at the origin of the artery which could be a site for reformation of thrombotic debris. The closure should be smooth and completely remove any stump of the internal carotid artery.

F. The distal end of the internal carotid artery is oversewn with 5/0 polypropylene. The primary arteriotomy is closed with continuous stitches of 6/0 polypropylene suture. The distal end of the suture line is started by passing both needles of the double-needle suture from the inside of the vessel and securing the suture by knot. The stitches are taken only a short distance from the edge of the arteriotomy on the external carotid artery to preserve maximum luminal diameter. Once onto the common carotid artery, more substantial stitches may be taken. Prior to final closure of the arteriotomy, the occlusion clamps are sequentially removed to flush out any air, clot, or debris to the arteriotomy.

G. The completed repair should appear as a smooth, continuous blood vessel from the common to the external carotid artery. Flow characteristics are monitored by Doppler ultrasound with the crystal applied directly to the vessel wall.

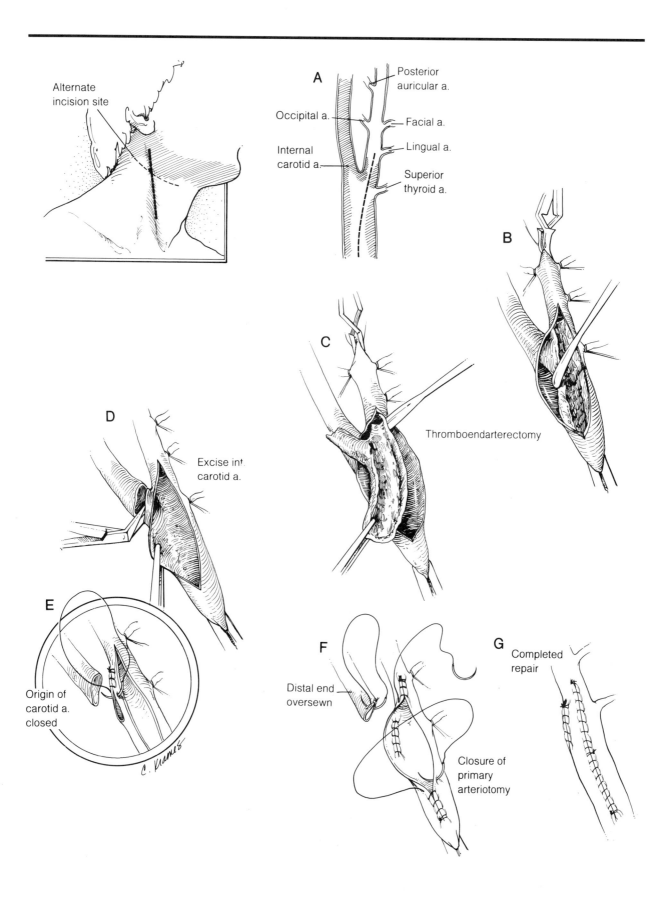

Alternate incision site

A

Posterior auricular a.

Occipital a.

Facial a.

Internal carotid a.

Lingual a.

Superior thyroid a.

B

C

Thromboendarterectomy

D

Excise int. carotid a.

E

Origin of carotid a. closed

C. KRAMES

F

Distal end oversewn

Closure of primary arteriotomy

G

Completed repair

Carotid Fibrodysplasia

4

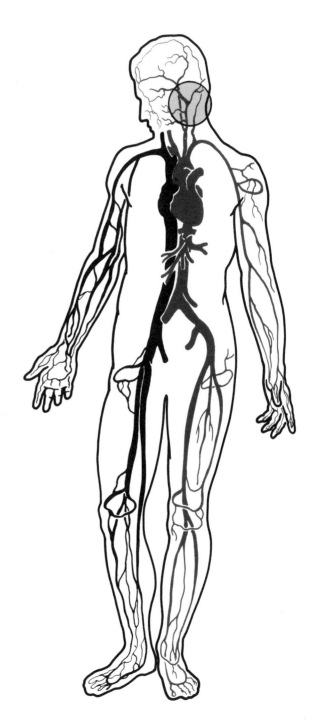

Fig 4–1. As for other operations on the carotid artery, fibrodysplasia of the internal carotid artery is approached by an incision paralleling the anterior border of the sterno-cleidomastoid muscle or the alternate skin line incision.

Fibrodysplasia of the internal carotid presents a typical angiographic pattern of irregular intimal surface that is easily recognized. The lesion involves the full thickness of the arterial wall and is not readily removed by endarterectomy. Dilation of the fibrotic artery will usually suffice to relieve stenosis.

A. The common carotid artery and its internal and external branches are exposed by usual dissection. Vascular clamps are applied to isolate the carotid bifurcation and the internal carotid artery. A shunt is not utilized in most cases. A short vertical arteriotomy is made in the common carotid artery near the bifurcation.

B. A peripheral vascular angioplasty catheter is passed through the arteriotomy into the internal carotid artery. This catheter has a volume-limited balloon attached to the distal end. The occlusion clamp is removed from the internal carotid artery so that the catheter may be passed beyond the distal limit of the fibrodysplastic changes in the vessel wall. The balloon is inflated to dilate the affected portion of the internal carotid artery. Formerly, olive-tipped metal dilators were passed through the stenotic artery to sequentially enlarge the lumen.

C. The arteriotomy is closed by continuous suture.

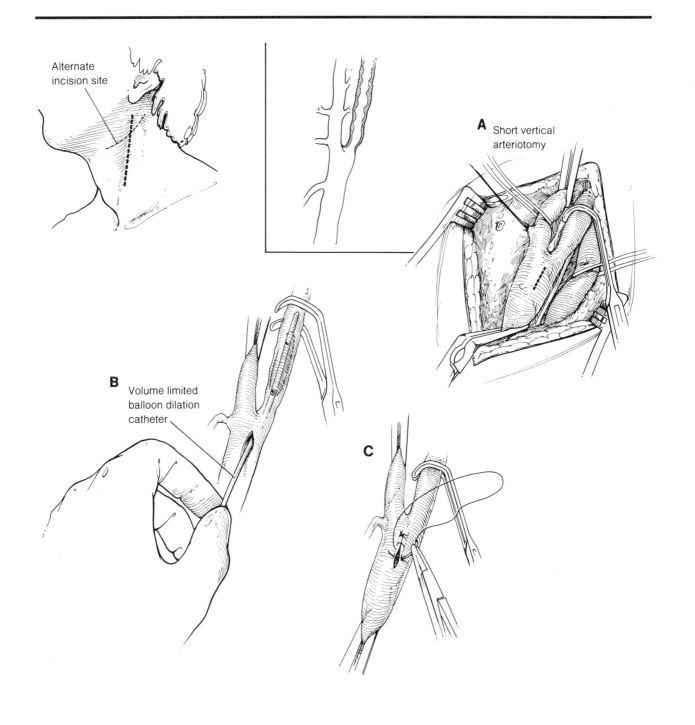

Alternate incision site

A Short vertical arteriotomy

B Volume limited balloon dilation catheter

C

Fig 4–2, A. Occasionally it may be necessary to resect the affected portion of the internal carotid artery. This is especially applicable where dilation techniques have failed to relieve stenosis. After complete mobilization of the carotid artery, vascular occlusion clamps are applied and the segment of abnormal internal carotid artery is excised.

B. The distal end of the carotid artery is enlarged by cutting back into the vessel wall (spatulation). An appropriate length of the greater saphenous vein is removed from the leg in the groin. It is beveled at the end and also cut back if necessary. An end-to-end anastomosis of the distal carotid artery to the saphenous vein graft is constructed by opposing the bevels of the vessels using two separate sutures to avoid any possibility of narrowing of the anastomosis. Continuous stitches of 6/0 polypropylene suture are used.

C. An anastomosis of the saphenous vein graft to the internal carotid artery origin is constructed by continuous suture to complete the repair.

D. A shunt catheter may be used to maintain cerebral blood flow to the distal carotid artery. The saphenous vein graft is placed over the shunt catheter prior to inserting the shunt and securing it proximally and distally with tourniquets.

E. An end-to-end anastomosis of the saphenous vein graft to the distal internal carotid artery is constructed with the shunt catheter acting as a stent. The posterior one-half of the proximal end-to-end anastomosis is constructed with the shunt in place.

F. The shunt is removed and the proximal anastomosis finished to complete the repair. Cerebral blood flow is restored through the interposed segment of saphenous vein graft.

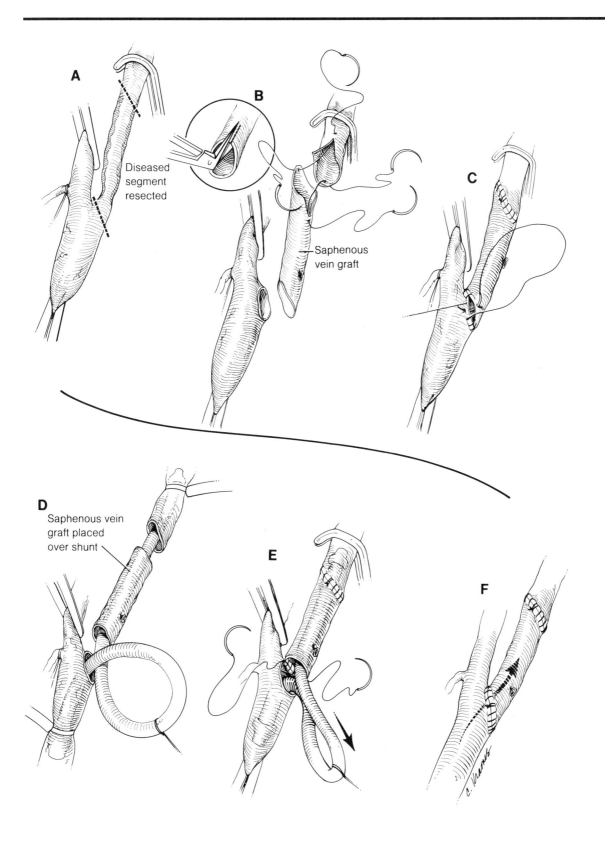

A

Diseased
segment
resected

B

Saphenous
vein graft

C

D

Saphenous vein
graft placed
over shunt

E

F

Carotid Aneurysm

5

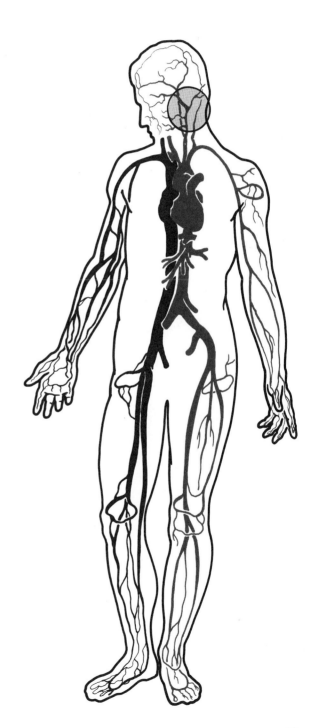

Aneurysm of Internal Carotid Artery

Fig 5–1. Aneurysm involving the internal carotid artery is treated by resection and interposition of saphenous vein graft. The lesion is approached through an incision that parallels the anterior border of the sternocleidomastoid muscle. The incision is taken higher on the neck than for other carotid operations because the control of the internal carotid artery distal to the aneurysm is often difficult.

A. The aneurysm is separated from the external carotid artery. Vascular control is obtained on the common carotid artery and the external and internal branches of the artery. The superior thyroid artery is controlled by loop ligature. The internal jugular vein is mobilized laterally. Dissection is taken superiorly enough to control the internal carotid artery distal to the aneurysm.

B. Vascular clamps are applied to isolate the lesion. The operation is usually performed without internal shunting unless there is marked change in the electroencephalogram which is monitored continuously. The aneurysm is opened longitudinally to accurately visualize the transition to normal internal carotid artery at the distal end. The artery is transected at that point and the aneurysm resected back to the origin of the internal carotid artery. The internal carotid artery is transected proximally by angulated incision into the carotid bulb.

C. The internal carotid artery is cut back slightly to enlarge the circumference available for anastomosis.

D. A segment of the greater saphenous vein is removed from the groin. The slightly beveled end of the vein graft is anastomosed in end-to-end fashion to the internal carotid artery with 6/0 polypropylene suture. The opposite end of the saphenous vein graft is cut back (spatulated) to achieve a circumference for anastomosis that approximates the opening in the carotid bulb.

E. An anastomosis of the saphenous vein graft to the carotid artery proximally is performed using continuous stitches of 6/0 or 5/0 polypropylene suture depending on the thickness of the carotid artery. The initial five suture loops are placed at the cut back portion of the saphenous vein graft that lies next to the external carotid artery to assure accuracy of this critical point of the anastomosis.

F. The suture loops are pulled up and the anastomosis completed anteriorly.

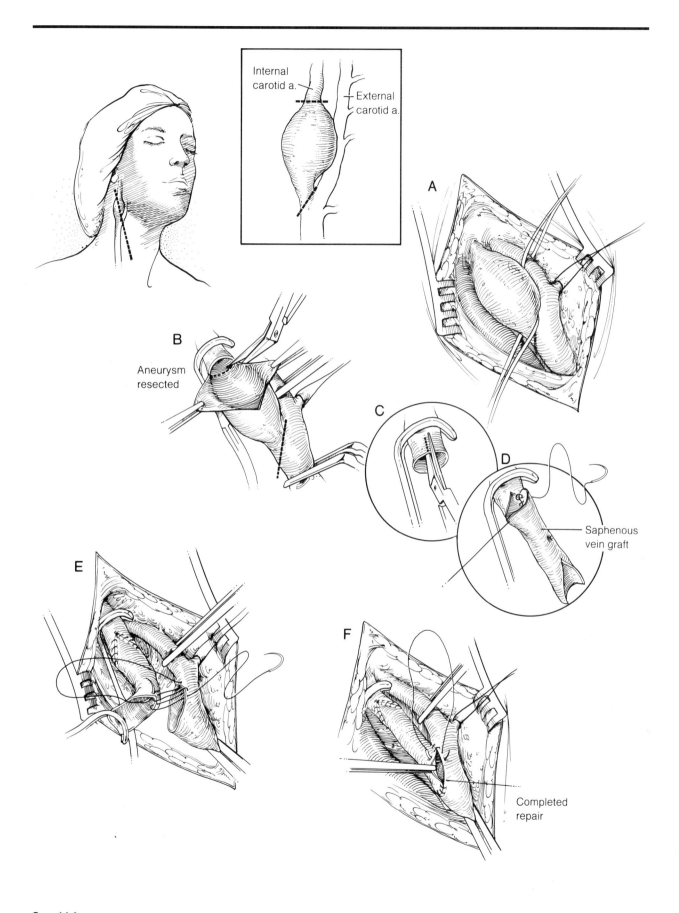

Internal carotid a.

External carotid a.

A

B

Aneurysm resected

C

D

Saphenous vein graft

E

F

Completed repair

Aneurysm With Tortuous Internal Carotid Artery

Fig 5–2. Tortuousity of the internal carotid artery may be associated with aneurysm of the artery. The extra length of the artery may make possible resection with end-to-end anastomosis of the artery.

A. The common carotid artery with the internal and external branches are completely mobilized. The aneurysm is resected by dividing the internal carotid artery at the edges of the aneurysm.

B. The internal carotid artery is mobilized superiorly to obtain sufficient length to approximate the ends. An end-to-end anastomosis is constructed by continuous stitches of 6/0 polypropylene suture.

C. The anastomosis is completed, restoring continuity of the internal carotid artery.

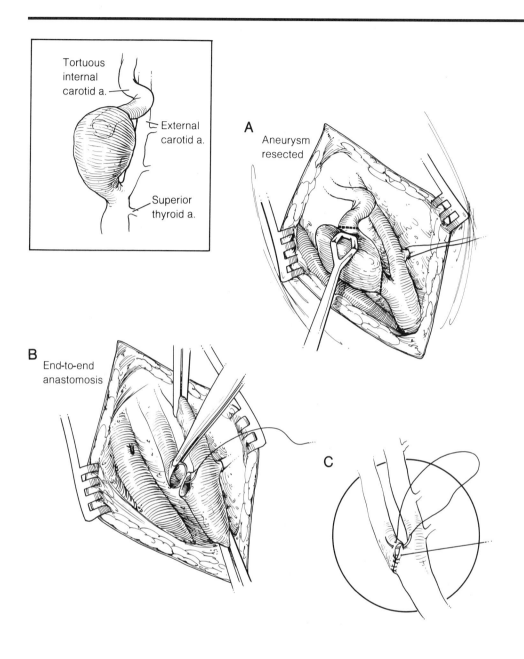

Tortuous
internal
carotid a.

External
carotid a.

Superior
thyroid a.

A Aneurysm
resected

B End-to-end
anastomosis

C

Aneurysm of the Carotid Artery Bifurcation

Fig 5–3. Aneurysm involving the bifurcation of the carotid artery is treated by resection and reconstruction using saphenous vein graft. The arteries are divided at the entry point to the aneurysm.

A. The common carotid artery, the aneurysm, and the internal and external branches of the artery are mobilized and controlled. The internal jugular vein is mobilized laterally. The superior thyroid artery is controlled by loop ligature.

B. Vascular clamps are applied to isolate the aneurysm. The internal and external carotid arteries are divided. The internal carotid artery is cut back slightly to create a greater circumference for anastomosis. The aneurysm is opened longitudinally to accurately visualize the junction of the normal common carotid artery. The artery is divided at that point and the aneurysm removed.

C. Since the reconstruction is complex and consumes considerable time, a shunt catheter is used to supplement cerebral blood flow. The catheter is inserted to the internal and common carotid arteries and held in place with tourniquets. A segment of saphenous vein taken from the groin is placed over the shunt catheter prior to insertion of the shunt.

D. An end-to-end anastomosis of the slightly beveled saphenous vein graft is made to the cut back internal carotid artery using 6/0 polypropylene suture. A longitudinal incision is made into the vein graft at a point that approximates the location of the external carotid artery. An end-to-side anastomosis of the external carotid artery to the vein graft is constructed using 6/0 polypropylene suture.

E. An end-to-end anastomosis of the common carotid artery to the proximal end of the saphenous vein graft is constructed. The back half of the anastomosis is performed with the shunt catheter in place.

F. The shunt catheter is removed through the proximal anastomosis, and occlusion clamps are applied to the common carotid artery and the internal carotid artery. A previously placed traction suture on the shunt catheter aids this maneuver.

G. The proximal anastomosis is completed and blood flow restored through the completed repair.

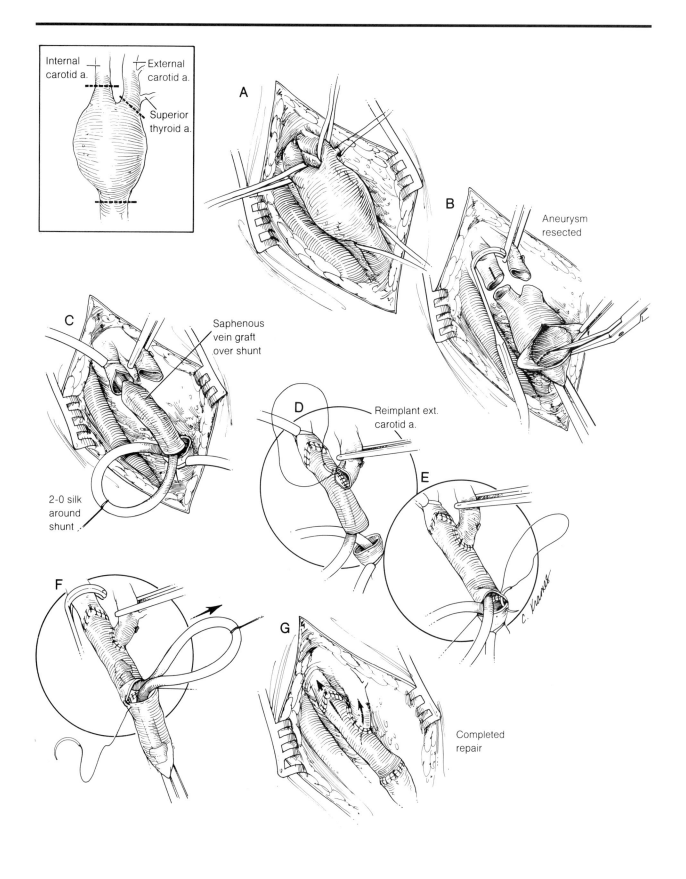

Internal carotid a.

External carotid a.

Superior thyroid a.

A

B

Aneurysm resected

C

Saphenous vein graft over shunt

2-0 silk around shunt

D

Reimplant ext. carotid a.

E

F

G

Completed repair

C. Vranes

Carotid Aneurysm

Carotid-subclavian Bypass

6

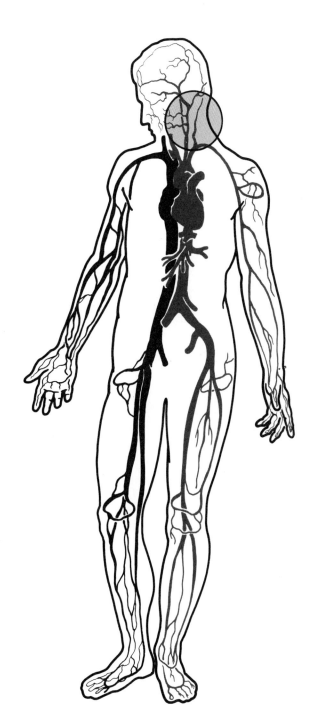

Carotid Artery Bypass

Fig 6–1. Bypass from the common carotid artery to the subclavian artery is performed for symptomatic occlusions of the subclavian artery that are proximal to the origin of the verterbral artery. When there are symptoms of verterbral-basilar insufficiency due to retro-flow of blood through the verterbral artery from the cerebral circuit to the arm, the condition is treated by utilizing carotid subclavian bypass.

A. The common carotid artery and the subclavian artery are approached through a skin line incision in the neck just above the clavicle. The incision is placed over the sternocleidomastoid muscle and extended slightly lateral to the clavicular head of that muscle. The clavicular head of the muscle is divided by cautery and retracted by self-retaining retractor.

B. The omohyoid muscle lies just below the sternocleidomastoid muscle. It is divided through its central tendinous portion.

C. The phrenic nerve is identified as it courses over the scalenus anticus muscle. The nerve is freed from the muscle and retracted. The scalenus anticus muscle is divided to gain access to the underlying vascular structures.

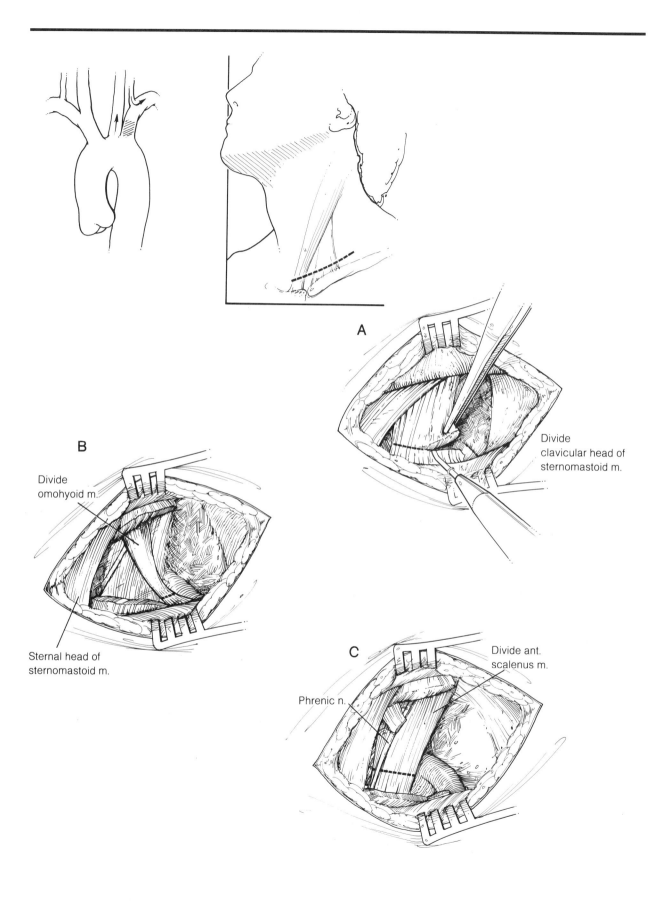

A

B

Divide
omohyoid m.

Sternal head of
sternomastoid m.

Divide
clavicular head of
sternomastoid m.

C

Divide ant.
scalenus m.

Phrenic n.

Carotid-subclavian Bypass

39

Fig 6–1, D. The internal jugular vein and common carotid artery are mobilized. The vagus nerve lies posterior and between these vessels and should be identified and preserved. The subclavian artery is identified and controlled with a vessel loop. It is mobilized sufficiently to allow good control. A portion of the subclavian vein will also be mobilized to provide access to the subclavian artery. Care is taken to identify and avoid injury to the thoracic duct. If it is inadvertently injured, it should be securely ligated to prevent a lymph fistula.

E. A curved vascular clamp (Derra) is used to isolate a segment of the common carotid artery. A longitudinal incision is made into the artery. The internal jugular vein is retracted laterally.

F. An 8-mm tubular prosthesis is beveled appropriately. An end-to-side anastomosis of the graft to the carotid artery is performed. Polypropylene suture is used (4/0 or 5/0). Continuous suture technique is utilized with the initial five suture loops placed at the heel of the graft prior to approximation of the graft to the artery.

G. Following completion of the graft to carotid artery anastomosis, the occlusion clamp is removed from the artery and a graft occlusion clamp (Fogarty) placed so as to restore carotid artery blood flow. The graft is taken posterior to the internal jugular vein. A curved vascular clamp (Derra) is used to isolate a segment of the subclavian artery. A longitudinal arteriotomy is made. The graft is shortened to correct length and beveled to appropriate angle for approximation to the subclavian artery. An end-to-side anastomosis of the graft to the subclavian artery is performed. Polypropylene suture (4/0 or 5/0) is used in continuous fashion placing the initial five suture loops around the heel of the graft prior to approximating graft and artery.

The completed bypass graft allows blood to flow from the carotid artery to the arm circulation rather than stealing from the posterior cerebral circulation via the vertebral artery. The incision is closed in layers by approximating the platysma muscle, superficial fascia, and skin leaving other muscles divided.

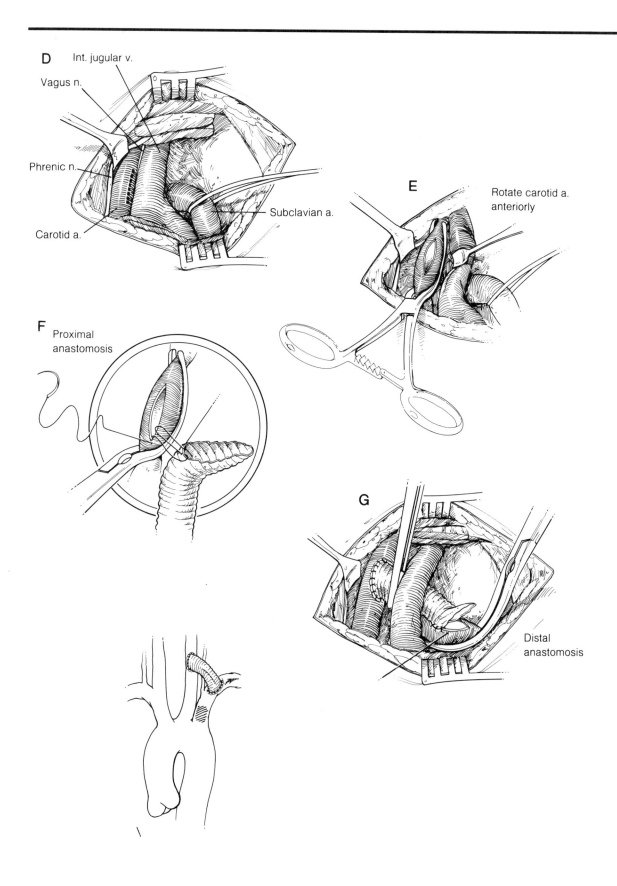

D

Int. jugular v.

Vagus n.

Phrenic n.

Carotid a.

Subclavian a.

E

Rotate carotid a. anteriorly

F Proximal anastomosis

G

Distal anastomosis

Carotid-Subclavian Bypass Combined With Carotid Endarterectomy

Fig 6–2. Proximal occlusion of the subclavian artery with subclavian steal syndrome due to retroflow of blood from the posterior cerebral circulation through the vertebral artery in conjunction with stenosis of the internal carotid artery requires combined treatment because simple common carotid-subclavian bypass could deprive the anterior cerebral circulation of sufficient flow. Two incisions are made. A skin line incision above the clavicle beginning over the sternocleidomastoid muscle and extending to the supraclavicular fossa laterally provides access to the subclavian artery. An incision parallel to the anterior border of the sternocleidomastoid to the angle of the mandible provides access to the carotid bifurcation.

A. Through these incisions, the common, external, and internal carotid arteries are mobilized. The internal jugular vein is mobilized more completely than for usual carotid endarterectomy. The clavicular head of the sternocleidomastoid muscle is divided near the clavicle to gain access to the subclavian artery. This artery is mobilized and controlled.

B. Vascular clamps are applied and standard carotid endarterectomy performed.

C. A tubular (8-mm diameter) vascular prosthesis is beveled appropriately to allow closure of the carotid arteriotomy by end-to-side anastomosis of graft to artery. The initial five suture loops at the heel of the graft are placed before approximating graft to artery.

D. Following completion of the graft-artery anastomosis, the occlusion clamps are removed from the carotid artery and a Fogarty clamp placed on the graft, thereby restoring cerebral blood flow. The graft is brought posterior to the internal jugular vein and behind the sternocleidomastoid muscle into the incision used to expose the subclavian artery. A segment of the subclavian artery is isolated by curved vascular clamp (Derra). Care is taken to avoid injury to the thoracic duct. A longitudinal arteriotomy is made to a length appropriate for the end of the vascular prosthesis. An end-to-side anastomosis of the graft to the subclavian artery is performed. Polypropylene suture (4/0 or 5/0) is used in continuous technique. Since the end of the graft in this circumstance is nearly straight or only slightly beveled, end-to-side technique is used in which the back wall of the anastomosis is performed first. This greatly facilitates exposure that may otherwise be difficult. The needles of the suture are passed inside-out on the artery and the graft at the proximal angle of the anastomosis. The needle on the graft side is then brought outside-in on the subclavian artery. The maneuver sets up the anastomosis so that suturing may be continued from the inside of the graft along the back side of the anastomosis.

The completed bypass graft not only enhances blood flow through the internal carotid artery to the cerebral circuit but also eliminates retro-flow through the posterior cerebral circulation through the verterbral artery by allowing flow from the common carotid artery through the graft to the subclavian artery.

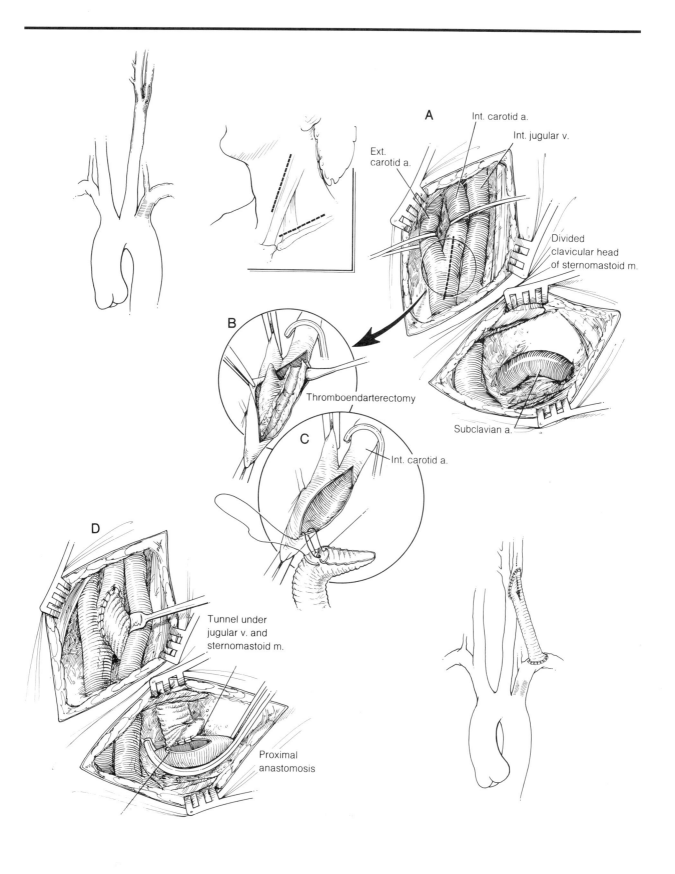

A

Ext.
carotid a.

Int. carotid a.

Int. jugular v.

Divided
clavicular head
of sternomastoid m.

B

Thromboendarterectomy

Subclavian a.

C

Int. carotid a.

D

Tunnel under
jugular v. and
sternomastoid m.

Proximal
anastomosis

Reimplantation of Carotid Artery

Fig 6–3. Stenosis of the left common carotid at its origin from the aortic arch can be treated by reimplantation of the common carotid artery to the subclavian artery, thereby avoiding thoracotomy which would be necessary to expose the area of stenosis. The operation is performed through a skin line incision just above the clavicle beginning over the sternocleidomastoid muscle and extending into the supraclavicular fossa.

A. The clavicular head of the sternocleidomastoid muscle and the scalenus anticus muscle are divided, preserving the phrenic nerve. The common carotid artery, internal jugular vein, and left subclavian artery are mobilized, with care to avoid injury of the thoracic duct. The vagus nerve is identified and preserved.

B. A vascular clamp (Derra) is placed on the common carotid artery in as proximal a location as possible. The artery is occluded distally and then divided.

C. The proximal end of the common carotid artery is oversewn with 5/0 polypropylene suture. The distal end of the carotid artery is drawn beneath the internal jugular vein to approximate the subclavian artery.

D. An end-to-side anastomosis of the common carotid artery to the subclavian artery is performed. The subclavian artery is isolated by curved vascular clamp and a longitudinal incision made into it. The anastomosis is made in usual nonbeveled end-to-side fashion by constructing the back side of the anastomosis working from within the arteries.

The completed anastomosis allows bypass of the proximal carotid artery stenosis and restores good cerebral blood flow via the left subclavian artery.

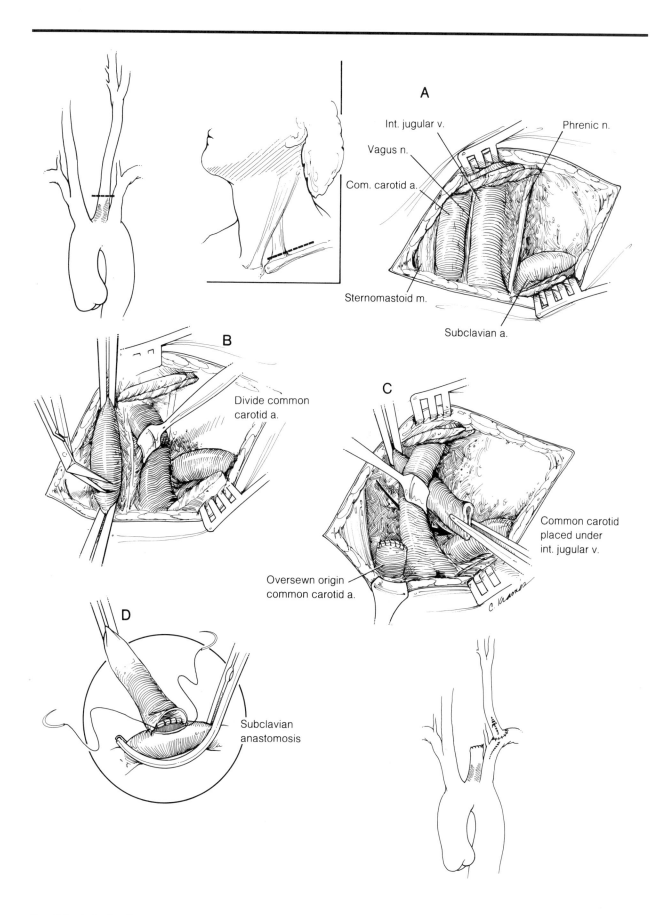

A

Int. jugular v.

Vagus n.

Com. carotid a.

Phrenic n.

Sternomastoid m.

Subclavian a.

B

Divide common carotid a.

C

Common carotid placed under int. jugular v.

Oversewn origin common carotid a.

D

Subclavian anastomosis

Aortic Arch Occlusive Disease

7

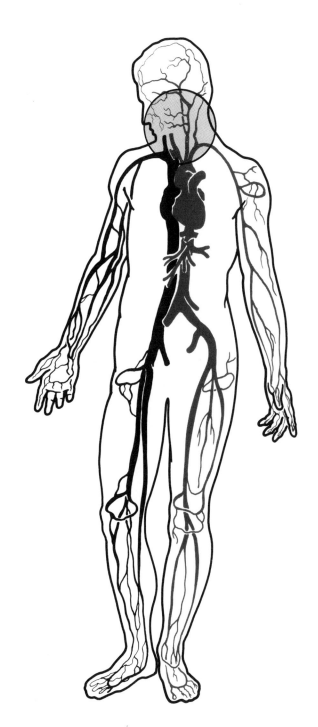

Endarterectomy of Aortic Origin of Innominate or Carotid Artery

Fig 7–1. Occlusive disease of the arterial branches of the aortic arches may be approached directly by thoracotomy or treated by extra-anatomic bypass grafts. Localized stenosis of the origin of the right brachiocephalic (innominate) artery or the origin of the left common carotid artery may be treated by performing endarterectomy of the obstructing plaque.

A midsternal incision is made. The incision is extended into the neck on the affected side.

A. The thymus is excised and the left innominate vein mobilized. The upper portion of the pericardium is opened to expose the aorta. The dissection proceeds superiorly over the aorta above the pericardial reflection to expose the innominate (or left common carotid) artery. The innominate artery is completely mobilized. The left innominate vein must be completely freed from the artery so that it may be retracted superiorly or inferiorly as the dissection proceeds. The right subclavian artery and the right common carotid artery are identified, mobilized, and controlled.

B. A curved vascular clamp (Lambert-Kay) is placed part way across the aorta at the origin of the innominate artery. The clamp must be placed deep onto the aorta so that the innominate plaque is completely encompassed by the clamp. The right subclavian and right carotid artery are occluded with vascular clamps to isolate the area of disease at the origin of the innominate artery. A longitudinal arteriotomy is made through the atherosclerotic plaque at the origin of the innominate artery and extended into normal artery distally.

C. A Freer septum elevator is used to separate the atherosclerotic plaque from the adventitia-media layer. The proximal end is cut off cleanly, and the distal end is fashioned to feather off to normal intima of the innominate artery.

D. The arteriotomy is closed by direct continuous stitch using 4/0 or 5/0 polypropylene suture.

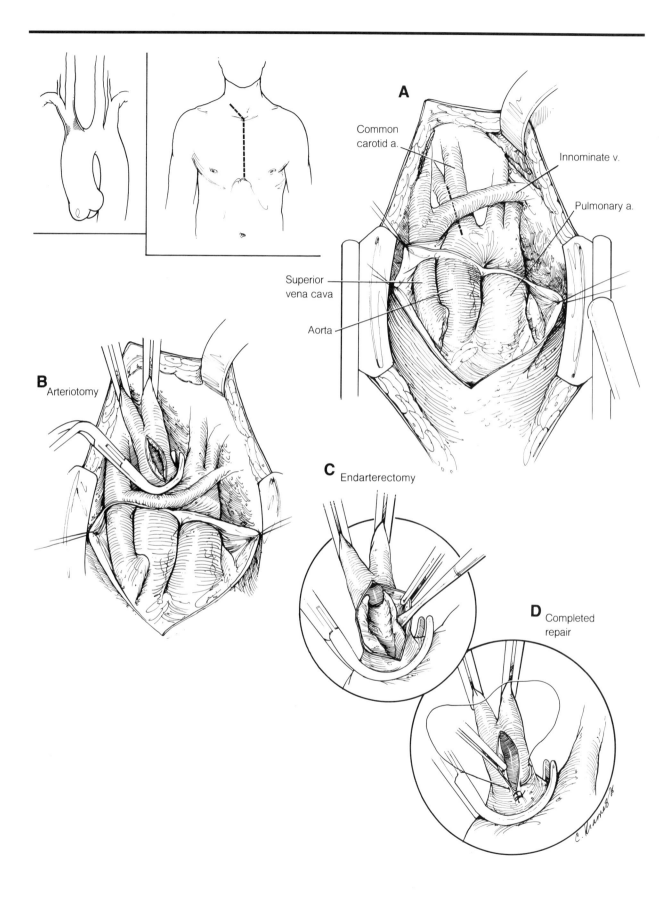

A

Common
carotid a.

Innominate v.

Pulmonary a.

Superior
vena cava

Aorta

B Arteriotomy

C Endarterectomy

D Completed
repair

Ascending Aorta—Carotid/Subclavian Artery Bypass

Fig 7–2. Occlusive disease involving most of the innominate artery is best treated using bypass technique rather than attempting primary treatment of the disease.

A midsternal incision is made with extension into the neck on the right side.

A. The upper portion of the pericardium is opened to expose the aorta. The left innominate vein is completely mobilized and freed from the underlying arteries. The dissection continues on the anterior surface of the aorta above the pericardial reflection. The right brachiocephalic (innominate) artery is identified. The dissection continues on the anterior surface of the innominate artery to its bifurcation. The right subclavian artery and the right common carotid artery are mobilized and controlled.

B. Vascular clamps are placed on the subclavian, carotid, and innominate arteries to isolate the innominate arterial bifurcation. The innominate artery is transected just below the bifurcation. The innominate vein is retracted inferiorly for exposure.

C. The proximal end of the innominate artery is closed by oversewing with 4/0 or 5/0 polypropylene.

D. A curved vascular clamp (Lambert-Kay) is used to partially occlude a convenient portion of the ascending aorta to isolate a portion of the aorta for the proximal anastomosis to the bypass graft. A longitudinal incision is made into the isolated portion of the aorta. An end-to-side anastomosis of a crimped tubular 10-mm diameter Dacron prosthesis is made to the aorta. Polypropylene suture material is used in 3/0 or 4/0 size depending on the characteristics of the aortic wall. The initial five suture loops at the heel of the graft are placed prior to approximating the graft to the aorta. The remainder of the anastomosis is constructed by continuous suture in usual fashion.

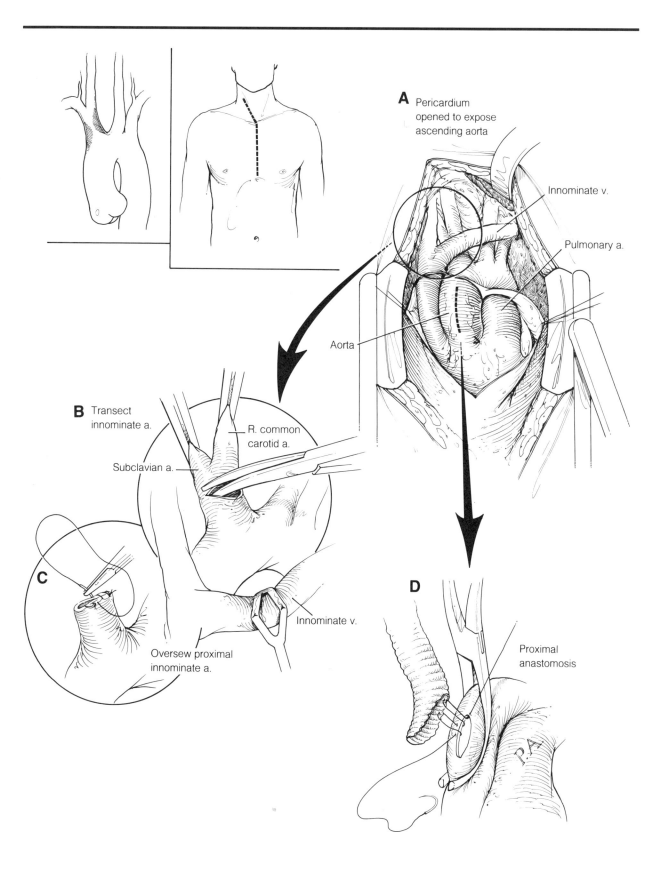

A Pericardium opened to expose ascending aorta

Innominate v.

Pulmonary a.

Aorta

B Transect innominate a.

R. common carotid a.

Subclavian a.

Innominate v.

C

Oversew proximal innominate a.

D Proximal anastomosis

P.A.

Fig 7–2, E. The vascular clamp is removed from the aorta and a soft-jaw clamp placed on the vascular graft. Hemostasis is secured at the proximal anastomosis. The vascular prosthesis is passed beneath the innominate vein or anterior to the vein, depending upon which pathway results in the least compression of the vein, and shortened appropriately to approximate the distal end of the innominate artery at the bifurcation. An end-to-end anastomosis is constructed by continuous stitch using 4/0 or 5/0 polypropylene depending on the thickness of the innominate artery. The suture loops of the back wall may be all placed before approximating graft to artery.

F. The completed repair shunts blood from the ascending aorta to the distal innominate artery through the vascular prosthesis.

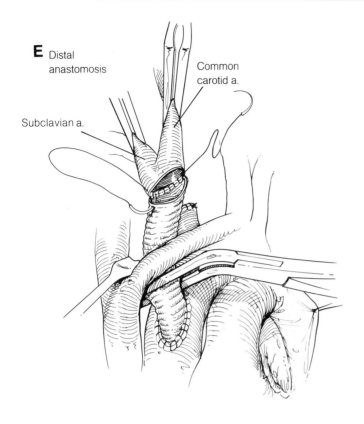

E Distal anastomosis

Subclavian a.

Common carotid a.

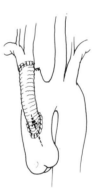

Ascending Aorta–Bilateral Carotid Artery Bypass

Fig 7–3. Proximal stenosis of the innominate artery and the left common carotid artery requires bilateral bypass to the carotid arteries to restore proper brain blood flow.

A midsternal incision is made with an extension into the neck on the right side. A second incision is made on the left side of the neck parallel to the anterior border of the sternocleidomastoid muscle.

A. The upper portion of the pericardium is opened to expose the aorta. The thymus is removed and the left innominate vein mobilized from the underlying arteries. The dissection is along the anterior surface of the innominate artery to the right common carotid artery. This artery is controlled in the neck. The left carotid artery bifurcation is mobilized. Incisions for bypass are made in the ascending aorta, the proximal portion of the right common carotid artery, and the left common carotid artery just below the bifurcation.

B. A bifurcated Dacron vascular prosthesis is used for the bypass graft. A 16 × 8-mm tubular prosthesis is usually about right, but the size actually chosen depends on the size of the common carotid arteries. The graft is beveled close to the bifurcation, leaving a short "heel" near the limb origins.

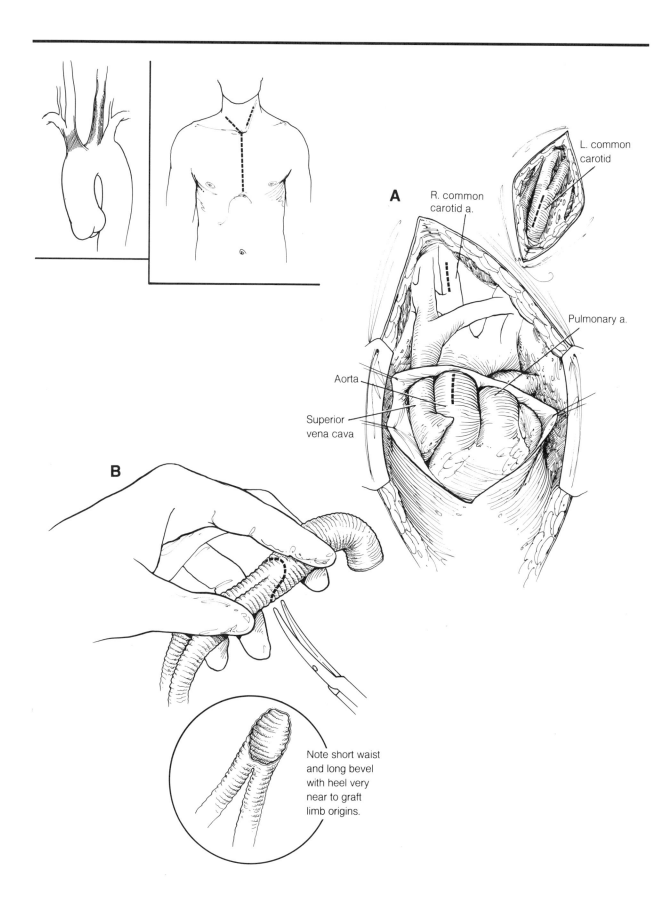

A

L. common carotid

R. common carotid a.

Pulmonary a.

Aorta

Superior vena cava

B

Note short waist and long bevel with heel very near to graft limb origins.

Fig 7–3, C. A curved vascular clamp (Lambert-Kay) is used to partially occlude the ascending aorta to exclude a portion of the anterior wall. A longitudinal arteriotomy is made in the ascending aorta. An end-to-side anastomosis of graft to the aorta is constructed by continuous stitch of 3/0 or 4/0 polypropylene. The initial five suture loops are placed at the heel of the graft prior to approximating the graft to the aorta.

D. The proximal anastomosis is completed in routine fashion. The limbs of the graft are then brought into the neck. The right side is simply brought through the primary exposure. The left side requires a tunnel to communicate the two wounds. End-to-side anastomoses of graft to the carotid arteries are then constructed. A curved vascular clamp may be used to isolate the portion of carotid artery for anastomosis or separate above and below clamps may be used. A longitudinal arteriotomy is made. The graft is anastomosed to the artery by continuous stitch of 4/0 or 5/0 polypropylene. The initial five suture loops at the heel of the graft are placed prior to approximation of graft to the artery. The remainder of the anastomosis is constructed by continuous suture technique.

The completed repair provides bypass of the proximal obstructions of the innominate and left common carotid artery via graft from ascending aorta to the common carotid arteries on right and left side of the neck.

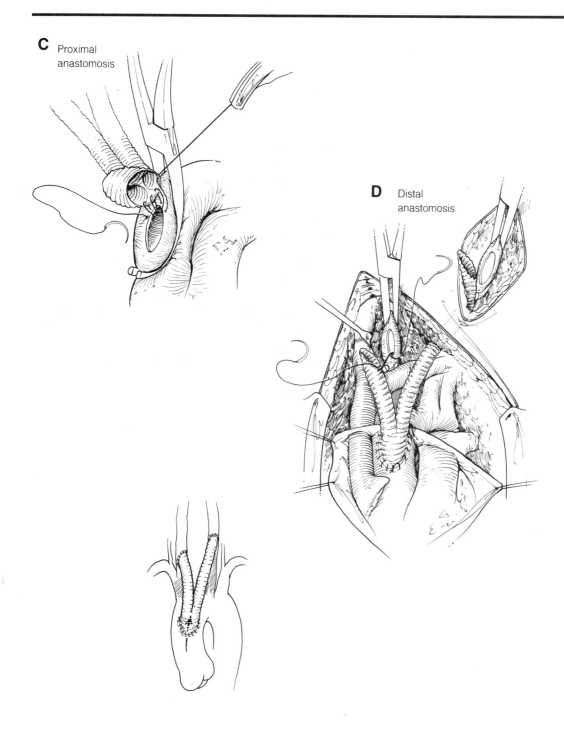

C Proximal anastomosis

D Distal anastomosis

Subclavian Artery–Internal Carotid Artery Bypass

Fig 7–4. Occlusion of the common carotid artery associated with stenosis of the internal carotid artery is treated utilizing bypass graft from the subclavian artery.

A. The exposure is that utilized for subclavian–carotid bypass using two incisions. One incision is above the clavicle in the supraclavicular fossa and the other parallel to the anterior border of the sternocleidomastoid muscle. The carotid bifurcation is mobilized and controlled. A longitudinal arteriotomy is made crossing the area of internal carotid stenosis into normal artery. A thromboendarterectomy is performed in the usual fashion using a Freer septum elevator.

B. The common carotid artery is divided a short distance below the bifurcation. The proximal carotid artery is closed by oversewing the vessel.

C. A segment of saphenous vein is removed from the groin and prepared for bypass graft in the usual fashion by ligating side branches and filling with solution to distend and test the vein graft. The vein graft is cut back to gain length for anastomosis. The end is fashioned to a point by excision of the edges of the vein graft. An end-to-end anastomosis of vein graft to the carotid artery is performed using continuous suture of 5/0 or 6/0 polypropylene. The "heel" of the vein graft is approximated to the "toe" of the artery. As usual, the initial five suture loops are placed around the heel of the vein graft prior to approximating the graft to the artery.

The bypass graft is completed by performing an end-to-side anastomosis of the vein graft to the subclavian artery.

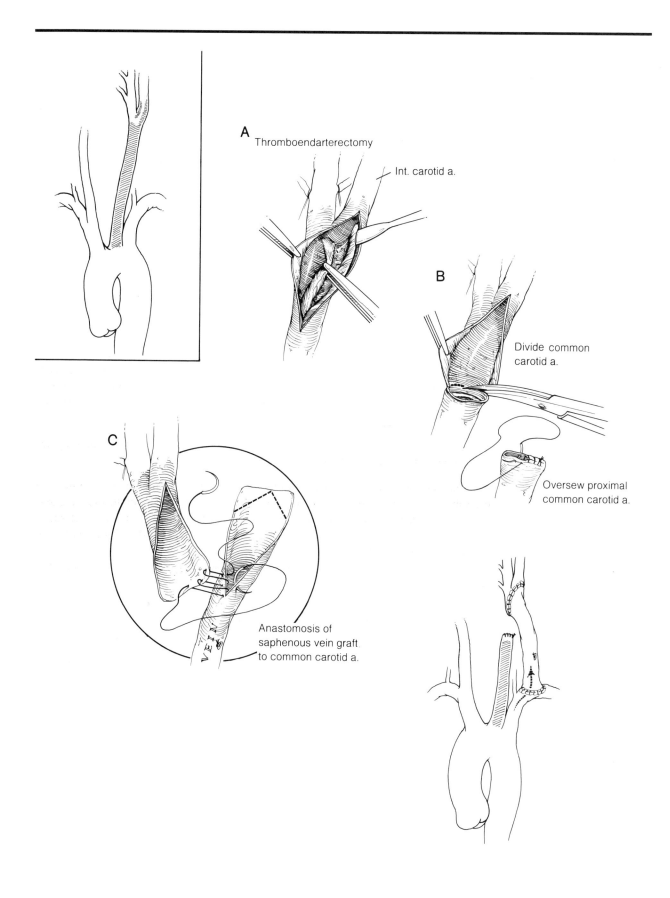

A Thromboendarterectomy

Int. carotid a.

B

Divide common carotid a.

Oversew proximal common carotid a.

C

Anastomosis of saphenous vein graft to common carotid a.

VEIN

Subclavian Artery–External Carotid Artery Bypass

Fig 7–5. Occlusion of the common and internal carotid artery with patent external carotid artery may also be amenable to bypass graft procedure using the subclavian artery as the proximal anastomosis and input to the graft.

A. The exposure is through two incisions in the neck. One incision is above and parallel to the clavicle and the other parallel to the anterior border of the sternocleidomastoid muscle. The carotid artery bifurcation is mobilized and dissection taken well up onto the external carotid artery controlling all side branches with loop ligatures. A light weight vascular clamp (Diethrich) is used to occlude the external carotid artery distally. An endarterectomy of the external carotid artery and a short segment of the internal carotid artery is performed.

B. The occluded internal carotid artery is ligated and excised from the common carotid artery at its origin.

C. The common carotid artery is divided just below the bifurcation.

D. A segment of saphenous vein is removed from the groin. The vein is prepared for bypass grafting in the usual fashion. The end of the vein graft is cut back to gain sufficient length for anastomosis. An end-to-end anastomosis of the vein graft to the carotid artery is constructed using 5/0 or 6/0 polypropylene suture material. The initial five stitches are placed at the heel of the graft to approximate it to the toe of the artery prior to bringing the vein graft into contact with the artery.

E. The anastomosis is completed using continuous stitches of 5/0 or 6/0 polypropylene depending on the thickness of the carotid artery.

F. The vein graft is taken posterior to the jugular vein and brought in proximity with the subclavian artery. An end-to-side anastomosis of the vein graft to the subclavian artery is constructed using continuous stitches of 5/0 or 6/0 polypropylene. The subclavian artery is isolated with a single curved vascular clamp (Derra) and the anastomosis is to a longitudinal arteriotomy.

The completed repair shunts blood from the subclavian artery to the external carotid artery.

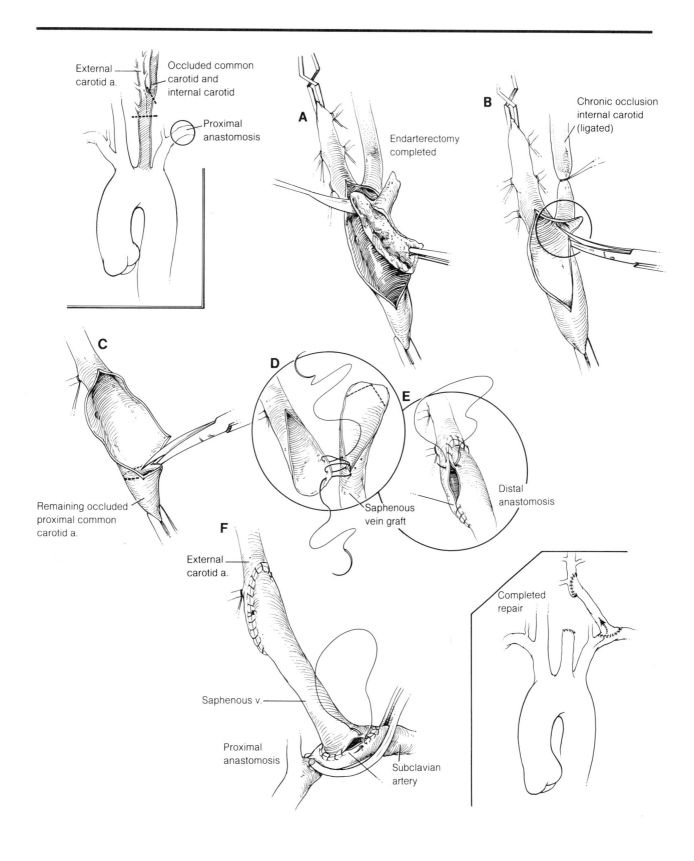

External carotid a.

Occluded common carotid and internal carotid

Proximal anastomosis

A

Endarterectomy completed

B

Chronic occlusion internal carotid (ligated)

C

D

E

Saphenous vein graft

Distal anastomosis

Remaining occluded proximal common carotid a.

F

External carotid a.

Saphenous v.

Proximal anastomosis

Subclavian artery

Completed repair

Subclavian Artery–Subclavian Artery Bypass

Fig 7–6. Stenosis or occlusion of the innominate artery may be simply treated by extra-anatomic bypass bringing blood from the contralateral subclavian artery across the neck to the ipsilateral subclavian artery.

The operation is performed through bilateral incisions above the clavicle in the supraclavicular fossa.

A. The clavicular head of the sternocleidomastoid muscle is divided.

B. The phrenic nerve lies on the anterior surface of the scaleneus anticus muscle. The nerve must be mobilized and protected to allow division of the anterior scalene muscle. The subclavian artery is exposed beneath the scalene muscle. Care is taken to avoid injury to the thoracic duct as it enters the subclavian vein-internal jugular vein confluence.

C. An end-to-side anastomosis of a prosthetic graft to the subclavian artery is performed. The subclavian artery is isolated with a single curved vascular clamp (Derra) so that a longitudinal arteriotomy may be made.

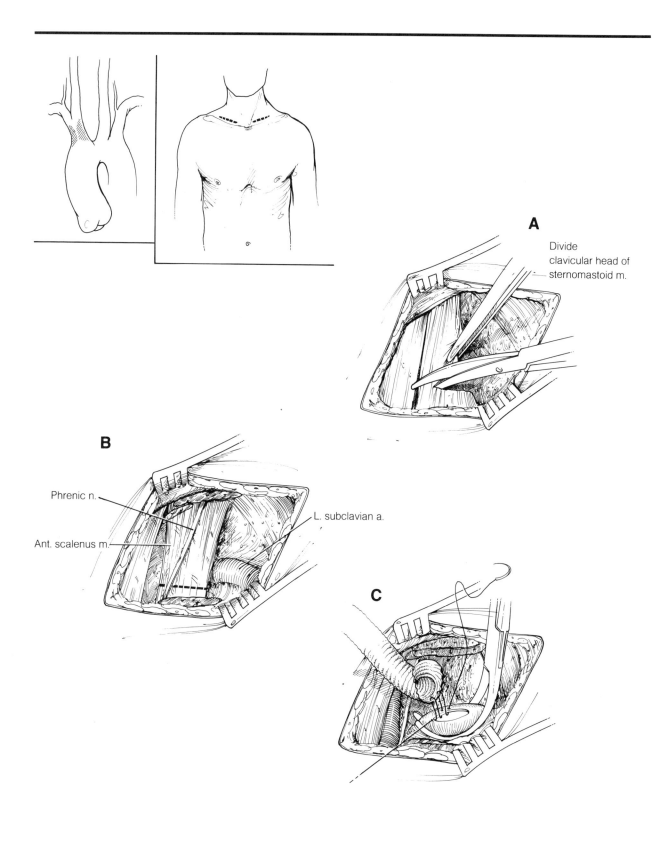

A

Divide clavicular head of sternomastoid m.

B

Phrenic n.

Ant. scalenus m.

L. subclavian a.

C

Fig 7–6, D. A tunnel is created in front of the internal jugular veins and behind the sternocleidomastoid muscle just above the sternum. The vascular graft is passed through the tunnel into the incision on the other side of the neck.

E. The subclavian artery is exposed and controlled in the same fashion as previously described. An end-to-side anastomosis of the graft to a longitudinal arteriotomy in the subclavian artery is performed using continuous stitches of 4/0 or 5/0 polypropylene.

The completed bypass graft brings blood from the subclavian artery on the unaffected side to the subclavian artery on the affected side.

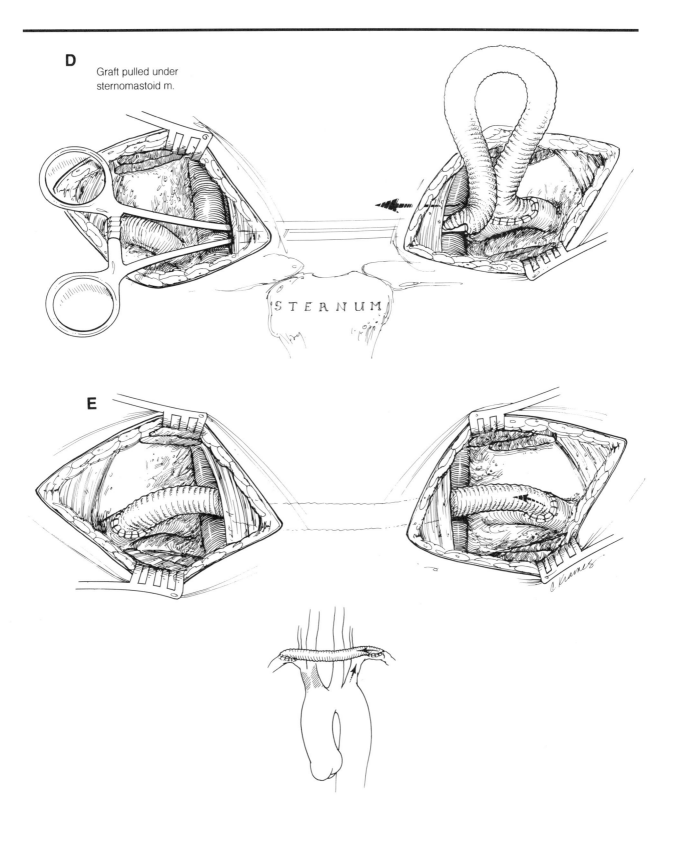

D

Graft pulled under
sternomastoid m.

STERNUM

E

Subclavian Artery–Bilateral Carotid Artery Bypass

Fig 7–7. Stenosis or occlusion of the innominate artery and the left common carotid artery may be treated by extra-anatomic bypass basing the input to the bypass graft on the left subclavian artery.

A collar incision is made low in the neck extending further into the supraclavicular fossa on the left side than on the right.

A. The left subclavian artery is exposed a little more lateral than usual for carotid-subclavian artery bypass. It may not be necessary to divide the clavicular head of the sternocleidomastoid muscle or the scaleneus anticus muscle. The subclavian artery is mobilized. The left common carotid artery is exposed and mobilized. An end-to-side anastomosis of an 8- or 10-mm diameter prosthetic graft to a longitudinal arteriotomy in the left subclavian artery is performed. Continuous stitches of 4/0 or 5/0 polypropylene are used. Placing the arteriotomy fairly lateral and making a significant bevel are necessary so that the graft will take a transverse orientation without kink after the anastomosis is made.

B. The graft is brought behind the mobilized sternocleidomastoid muscle and in front of the internal jugular vein. The left common carotid artery is mobilized and isolated by vascular clamp. Separation of the clavicular and sternal heads of the sternocleidomastoid muscle will aid exposure. A punch incision of the carotid artery will make the anastomosis easier to perform and may be more reliable than longitudinal arteriotomy. A side-to-side anastomosis of the graft to the common carotid artery is performed using continuous stitches of 4/0 or 5/0 polypropylene. A real effort should be made to keep the anastomosis low in the neck and just above the sternum and clavicles.

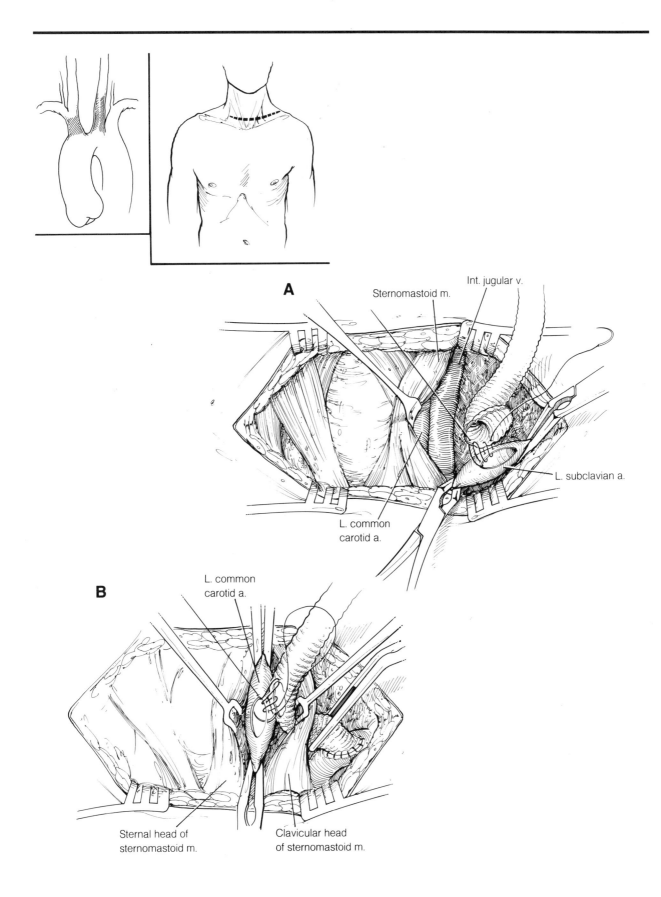

A

Int. jugular v.

Sternomastoid m.

L. common
carotid a.

L. subclavian a.

B

L. common
carotid a.

Sternal head of
sternomastoid m.

Clavicular head
of sternomastoid m.

Fig 7–7, C. The vascular clamps are removed from the left common carotid artery and a soft jaw clamp (Fogarty) placed on the graft so that cerebral blood flow may be established from the left subclavian artery and graft to the left carotid artery. The graft is brought across the midline in front of the trachea. The right sternocleidomastoid muscle is retracted to expose the right common carotid artery. It may be best to separate the clavicular and sternal heads of that muscle to gain access to the artery. The right common carotid artery is mobilized and controlled with a single curved vascular clamp. An end-to-side anastomosis of the graft to a punch arteriotomy in the carotid artery is performed. Continuous stitches of 4/0 or 5/0 polypropylene are used.

Opening the bypass graft restores blood flow to the carotid arteries and the right subclavian artery with the input to the graft from the left subclavian artery.

C

R. common
carotid a.

L. common
carotid a.

Int. jugular v.

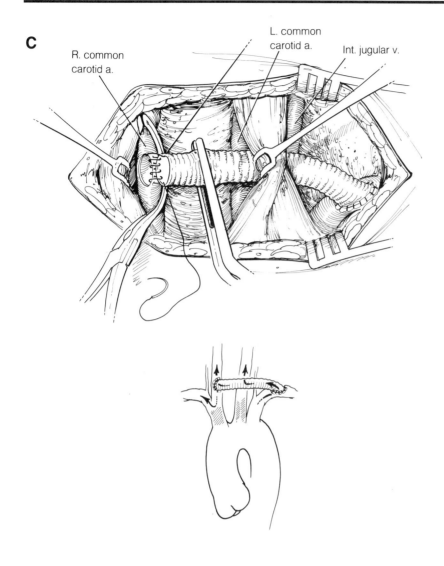

Carotid Body Tumor

8

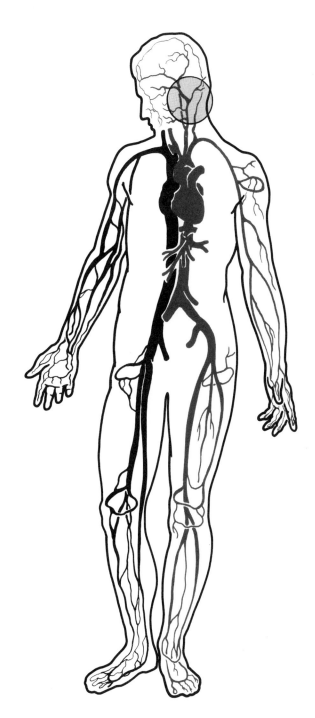

Fig 8–1. Carotid body tumor presents as a pulsatile mass in the neck in the region of the carotid bifurcation. Angiography confirms the presence of a highly vascular tumor above the carotid bifurcation which displaces both the internal and external carotid arteries. Presence of the lesion is indication for resection. The operation is performed through an incision in the neck which parallels the anterior border of the sternocleidomastoid muscle extending near to the angle of the mandible. The groin and thigh of the patient are prepared in case a segment of saphenous vein is required for the reconstruction.

A. The tumor is freed from the sternocleidomastoid muscle. The common carotid artery is dissected free of the vagus nerve and the internal jugular vein, which is retracted laterally. Dissection is taken cephalad to mobilize the internal and external carotid arteries along with the tumor mass which is in the carotid bifurcation. Branches of the external carotid artery are ligated and divided.

B. The most common complication of resection of carotid body tumor is injury to the hypoglossal nerve. This nerve should be identified and dissected away from the tumor. Finger retraction downward on the tumor mass will allow exposure of the hypoglossal nerve which is then dissected free and protected from injury.

C. Carotid body tumors are extremely vascular. Profuse bleeding occurs if the capsule of the tumor is opened. The resection of the tumor proceeds in the adventitial plane of the internal carotid artery. The adventitial tissue plane is established in the common carotid artery and continued into the internal carotid artery. Sharp dissection with scissors is used.

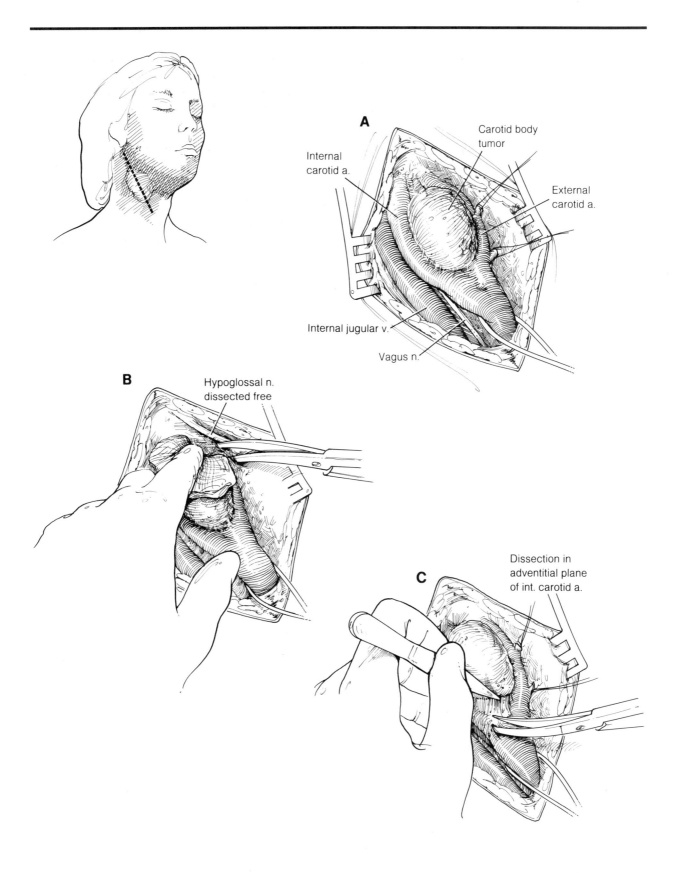

A

Internal carotid a.

Carotid body tumor

External carotid a.

Internal jugular v.

Vagus n.

B

Hypoglossal n. dissected free

C

Dissection in adventitial plane of int. carotid a.

Fig 8–1, D. The tumor is patiently separated from the internal carotid artery. The dissection is continued to the upper extent of the tumor. The hypoglossal nerve is separated completely from the tumor. The nerve of the carotid body is divided. Any bleeding points in the media of the internal carotid artery are repaired with 6/0 or 7/0 polypropylene.

E. The external carotid artery is ligated at the upper extent of tumor attachment. A vascular clamp is placed on the proximal external carotid artery. The external carotid artery is resected with the tumor. The proximal end of the external carotid artery is oversewn as close to the bifurcation as possible.

F. In some cases it is not possible to develop an adequate subadventitial place for resection of the tumor, and the internal carotid artery becomes damaged or must be removed with the tumor. In these cases, a segment of saphenous vein is removed from the thigh and interposed between the carotid bifurcation and the distal internal carotid artery. End-to-end anastomoses are constructed in usual fashion.

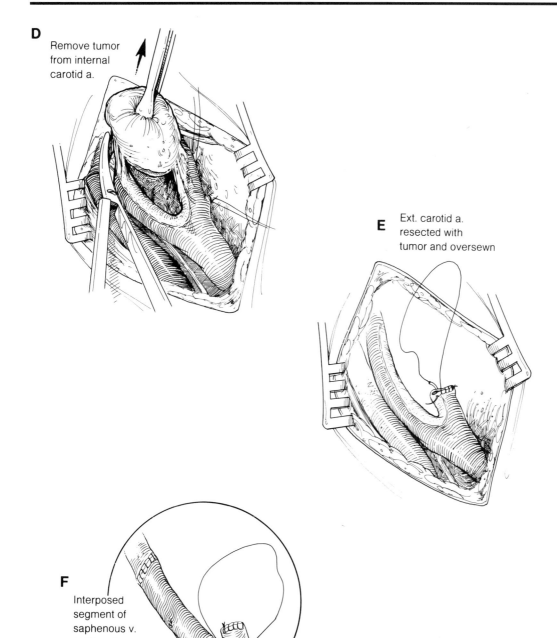

D

Remove tumor from internal carotid a.

E Ext. carotid a. resected with tumor and oversewn

F Interposed segment of saphenous v. graft

C. Kramer

Vertebral Artery
Revascularization

9

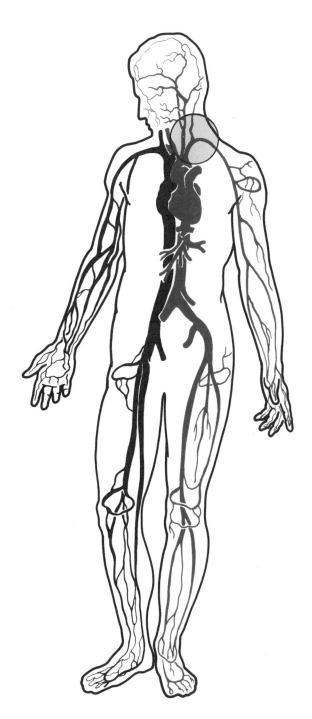

Fig 9–1. Stenosis of the origin of the vertebral artery in combination with other significant stenosis or occlusion of the contralateral vertebral artery and/or internal carotid artery may result in the syndrome of vertebral-basilar arterial insufficiency. These patients have dizziness, syncope, or facial numbness or weakness. Relief of arterial obstruction in the carotid arteries will usually relieve the syndrome, but there is an occasional patient in whom direct reconstruction of the vertebral artery is indicated.

The origin of the vertebral artery is approached through a skin line incision over the lateral aspect of the sternocleidomastoid muscle into the supraclavicular fossa just above the clavicle.

A. The subcutaneous tissues and the platysma muscle are divided. The clavicular head of the sternocleidomastoid muscle is divided.

B. The phrenic nerve is identified on the anterior surface of the scalenus anticus muscle. The nerve is mobilized and retracted so that the scalene muscle can be divided. This exposes the underlying subclavian artery. The artery is mobilized completely to expose the vertebral artery origin. It may be helpful to divide the thyrocervical trunk and the internal mammary artery. Care is taken to identify and avoid injury to the thoracic duct.

Subclavian–Vertebral Artery Vein Bypass Graft

A. A short segment of saphenous vein is removed from the leg. The end of the graft is beveled so that the graft will be properly oriented toward the vertebral artery after anastomosis. A segment of the subclavian artery is isolated by curved vascular clamp (Derra). An end-to-side anastomosis of the vein graft to the subclavian artery is constructed by usual technique.

B. A segment of the vertebral artery distal to the area of stenosis is isolated by curved vascular clamp. An incision is made into the artery. Loupe optical magnification (2.5–3.5×) is used to enhance visualization and accuracy of incision and anastomosis. An end-to-side anastomosis of the vein graft to the vertebral artery is constructed using continuous 6/0 or 7/0 polypropylene suture.

The completed repair provides blood flow to the distal vertebral artery through the bypass conduit from the subclavian artery.

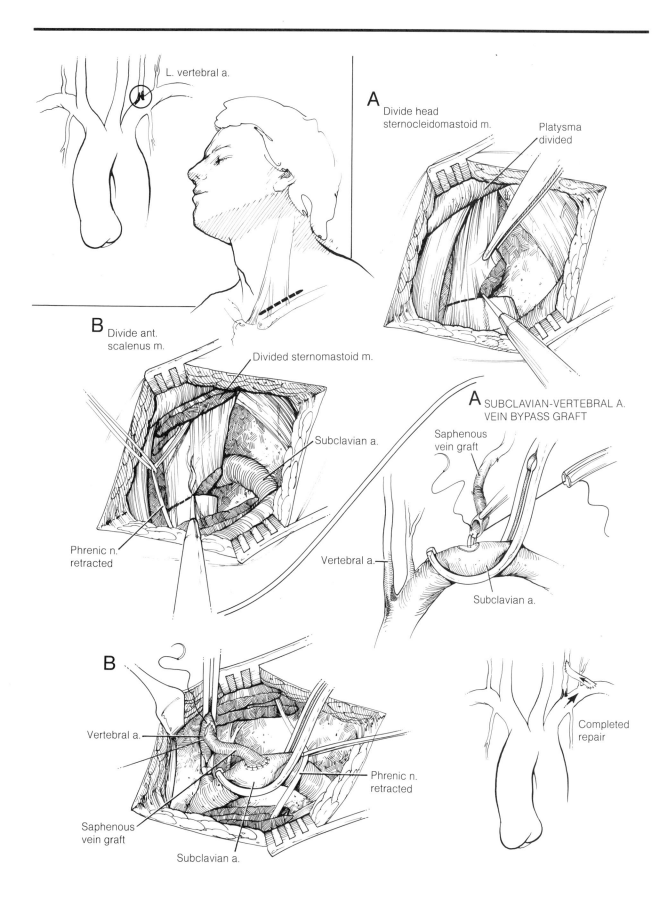

L. vertebral a.

A Divide head sternocleidomastoid m.

Platysma divided

B Divide ant. scalenus m.

Divided sternomastoid m.

Subclavian a.

Phrenic n. retracted

A SUBCLAVIAN-VERTEBRAL A. VEIN BYPASS GRAFT

Saphenous vein graft

Vertebral a.

Subclavian a.

B

Vertebral a.

Saphenous vein graft

Subclavian a.

Phrenic n. retracted

Completed repair

Implantation of Vertebral Artery to Common Carotid Artery

Fig 9–2. Proximal stenosis of the origin of the vertebral artery with satisfactory condition of the vessel wall distally may be treated by reimplantation of the artery to the adjacent common carotid artery.

A. Exposure must be more extensive with mobilization of the internal jugular vein, common carotid artery, and vertebral artery. The vein is retracted medially to expose the carotid artery. The vertebral artery is divided at its origin or just distal to the obstructing atherosclerotic plaque. The proximal end of the artery is oversewn. The distal end of the artery is cut back to provide a larger circumference for anastomosis. The common carotid artery is isolated by curved vascular clamp. A "round" arteriotomy is made using the Karp aortic punch. This type of arteriotomy assures that there will be no chance of collapse of the edges of the artery at the anastomosis. An end-to-side anastomosis of the verterbral artery to the common carotid artery is constructed by continuous suture technique using 5/0 or 6/0 polypropylene.

B. The completed anastomosis allows blood to flow directly to the verterbral artery from the carotid circulation.

Vertebral Endarterectomy

A. Localized plaques causing stenosis of the origin of the verterbral artery may be removed by endarterectomy. The origin of the vertebral artery and the surrounding subclavian artery must be mobilized completely. The vertebral artery origin is located on the posterior-superior aspect of the subclavian artery. The incision should begin in the subclavian artery and extend across the origin of the vertebral artery.

B. The subclavian artery on both sides of the vertebral artery is occluded using a single curved vascular clamp. The vertebral artery is occluded with a small vascular clamp (Diethrich). The incision is taken across the atherosclerotic plaque.

C. Endarterectomy is performed using the Freer septum elevator. The distal end of the dissection must achieve a smooth transition to the intima of the vertebral artery.

D. Closure of the arteriotomy displaces the origin of the vertebral artery to the superior surface of the subclavian artery. Each apex of the incision is approximated so that the incision is in effect closed transversely.

E. The completed closure brings the vertebral artery to a position more anterior on the subclavian artery.

F. An alternative approach is to place a vein patch into the arteriotomy. This widens out the origin of the vertebral artery and moves it more anterior on the subclavian artery.

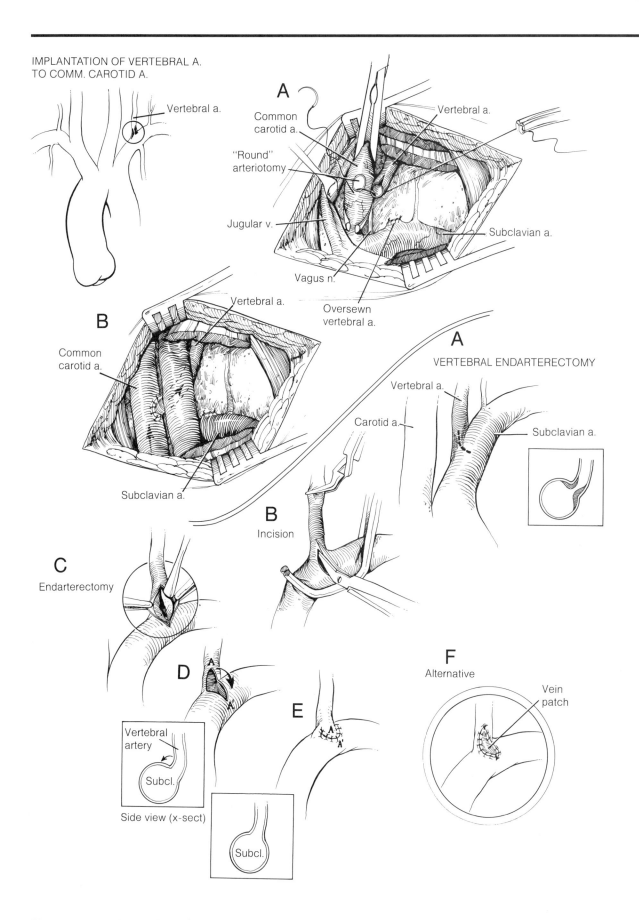

IMPLANTATION OF VERTEBRAL A.
TO COMM. CAROTID A.

Vertebral a.

A

Common
carotid a.

"Round"
arteriotomy

Jugular v.

Vertebral a.

Subclavian a.

Vagus n.

Oversewn
vertebral a.

B

Vertebral a.

Common
carotid a.

Subclavian a.

A

VERTEBRAL ENDARTERECTOMY

Vertebral a.

Carotid a.

Subclavian a.

B

Incision

C

Endarterectomy

D

Vertebral
artery

Subcl.

Side view (x-sect)

E

Subcl.

F

Alternative

Vein
patch

Subclavian-axillary Aneurysm

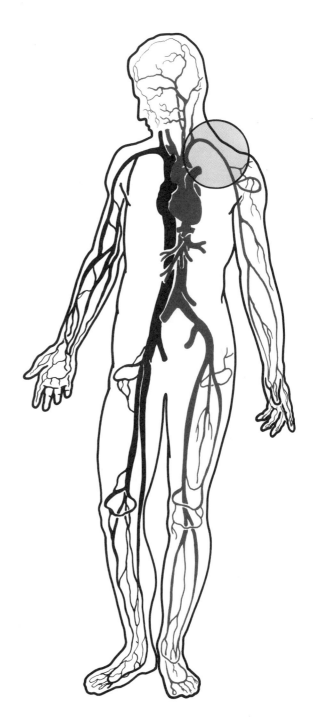

Subclavian Artery Aneurysm

Fig 10–1. Aneurysm of the subclavian artery located near the origin of the artery is an intrathoracic problem. It is best approached through the left pleural space via posterolateral thoracotomy through the fourth intercostal space.

A. The pleura over the upper portion of the descending thoracic aorta and left subclavian artery is incised. Retraction stitches are placed along the pleural edges to maintain exposure. The lung is retracted inferiorly. The aneurysm is exposed and freed from surrounding mediastinal tissue. Care is taken to avoid manipulation of the aneurysm as it will contain thrombus which can be easily embolized distally. Control of the subclavian artery proximal and distal to the aneurysm is obtained. The vagus and phrenic nerves should be identified and preserved.

B. Vascular clamps are applied to the subclavian artery proximal and distal to the aneurysm. A curved vascular clamp (Lambert-Kay or Cooley) is used proximally so that a portion of the aorta may be included in the clamp for more length on the subclavian artery at its origin.

C. The subclavian artery is divided proximal and distal to the aneurysm. The aneurysm is excised. Proximal and distal vessels are carefully inspected to be certain no thrombus from the aneurysm remains in the lumen.

D. A vascular graft is interposed between the ends of the subclavian artery. An end-to-end anastomosis of the graft to the distal subclavian artery is constructed by continuous suture of 4/0 polypropylene.

E. The proximal anastomosis to graft to artery is performed to complete the repair.

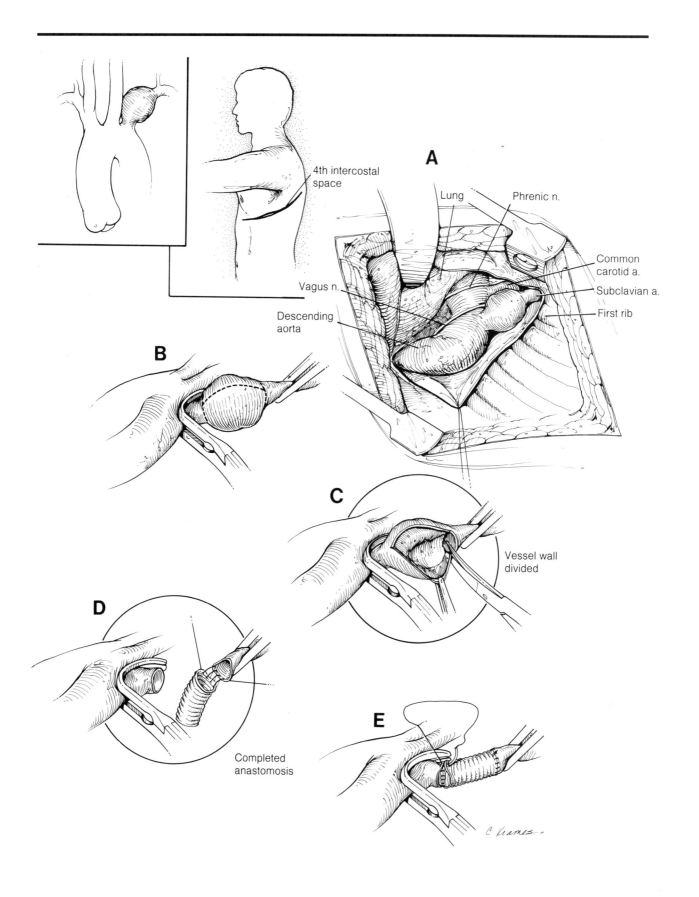

A

Lung

Phrenic n.

Common carotid a.

Subclavian a.

First rib

Vagus n.

Descending aorta

4th intercostal space

B

C

Vessel wall divided

D

Completed anastomosis

E

Axillary Artery Aneurysm

Aneurysm of the axillary artery may be approached outside the thorax provided it is assured that the most proximal portion of the aneurysm is beyond the edge of the first rib. An incision is made in the upper aspect of the anterior chest in the delto-pectoral groove across the clavicle to the pectoral fold below the head of the humerus. The arm is extended onto an arm board and prepared into the operating field.

Fig 10–1, F. The fibers of the pectoralis major muscle are separated. The pectoralis minor muscle is divided close to its tendon.

G. The aneurysm of the axillary artery is found near the clavicle as the artery emerges from the thorax over the first rib. The subclavian-axillary vein overlies the aneurysm and must be separated from it.

H. Vascular clamps are applied to the axillary artery proximal and distal to the aneurysm. The artery is divided and the aneurysm resected.

I. A vascular graft (6- to 8-mm diameter) is interposed between the ends of the axillary artery. An end-to-end anastomosis of graft to proximal artery is constructed. The distal anastomosis completes the repair.

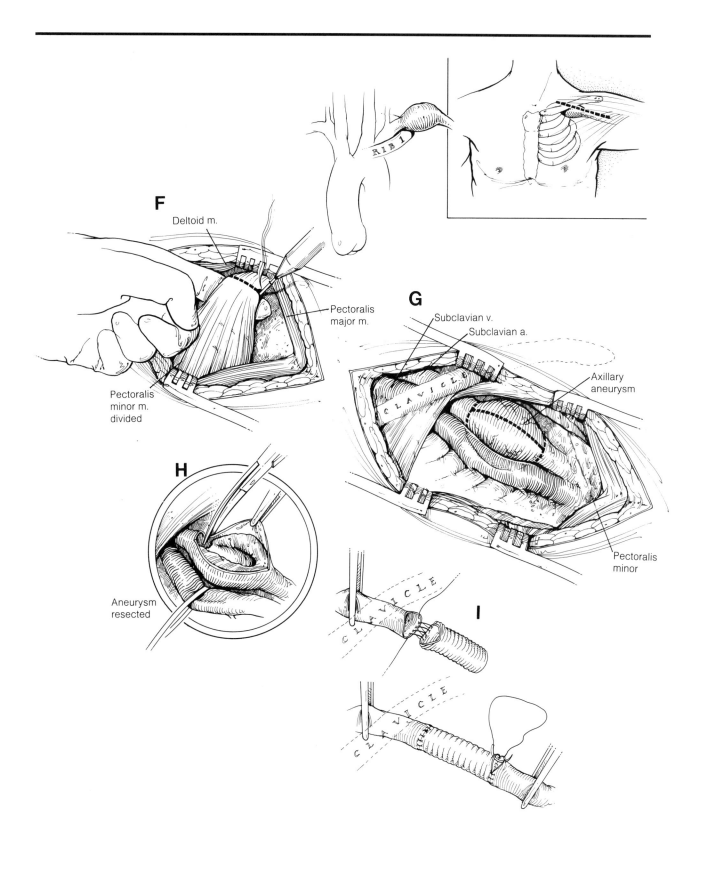

F

Deltoid m.

Pectoralis major m.

Pectoralis minor m. divided

G

Subclavian v.

Subclavian a.

Axillary aneurysm

Pectoralis minor

H

Aneurysm resected

I

11

Brachial-ulnar-radial
Artery Injuries

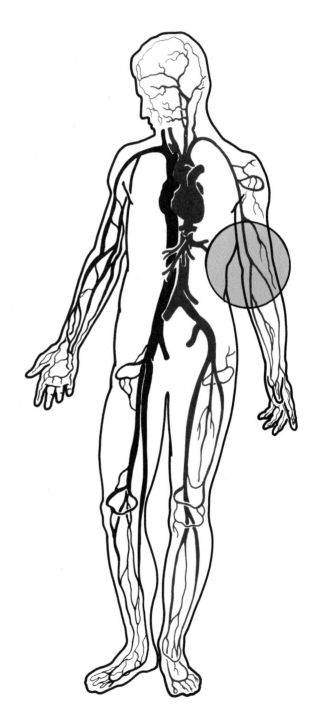

Fig 11–1. Reconstructive surgery for arteries of the arm is almost exclusively related to injury of these arteries. There are few degenerative conditions that affect arm arteries that require operative intervention. Since trauma often perforates the skin, the approach to the arteries of the arm may be determined in part by the location and extent of the injury on the skin.

A. The usual approach to the brachial artery is through a longitudinal incision on the medial aspect of the arm in the groove between the biceps and triceps muscles. Proximal control and exposure of the axillary artery is by proximal extension of the incision through the axilla and onto the chest wall in the delto-pectoral groove below the clavicle. This proximal extension creates a natural "S" as it crosses the lateral border of the pectoralis major muscle onto the chest wall. Distal exposure of the brachial artery and the origins of the radial and ulnar arteries in the antecubital fossa is by "S"-shaped incision from medial to lateral aspect of the arm across the elbow crease to avoid flexion contracture. Exposure of the radial artery is by longitudinal extension on the volar surface of the arm on the lateral aspect parallel to the radius and the course of the radial artery. Exposure of the ulnar artery is by longitudinal incision on the volar surface and medial aspect of the arm parallel to the ulna and ulnar artery.

B. The anatomy of the arm arterial circulation demonstrates the extensive opportunities for development of collateral pathways. The axillary artery passes beneath the pectoralis minor muscle into the axillary fossa. It continues into the arm as the brachial artery. The deep or profunda brachial artery takes origin in a somewhat variable position high in the upper arm. The deep brachial artery is connected to the radial and ulnar arteries by multiple arterial pathways around the elbow. In addition, the brachial artery is connected to the radial and ulnar arteries by existing collateral arteries at the elbow. Interruption of the brachial artery, therefore, is rarely associated with ischemia of arterial circulation to the hand. The radial and ulnar arteries take origin from the brachial artery at the elbow joint in the antecubital fossa. The deep circulation of the forearm is duplicated with the interosseous artery taking origin from the ulnar artery and dividing to form the volar and dorsal interosseous arteries placed anterior and posterior to the interosseous membrane. Deep circulation communicates with the radial and ulnar arteries at the wrist. The circulation in the hand is duplicated similarly with the presence of the dorsal and volar arches which communicate the digital arterial circulation.

C. Cross-sectional anatomy at mid-arm above the elbow demonstrates the close proximity of the median nerve to the brachial artery. It lies antero-medial to the artery. The ulnar nerve is not far posterior to the brachial artery and more medial than the median nerve.

D. Similarly, the cross-section of the arm below the elbow shows the close association of the radial and ulnar nerves to the respective artery. The interosseous membrane courses between the radius and ulna with volar and dorsal interosseous arteries on each side of the membrane.

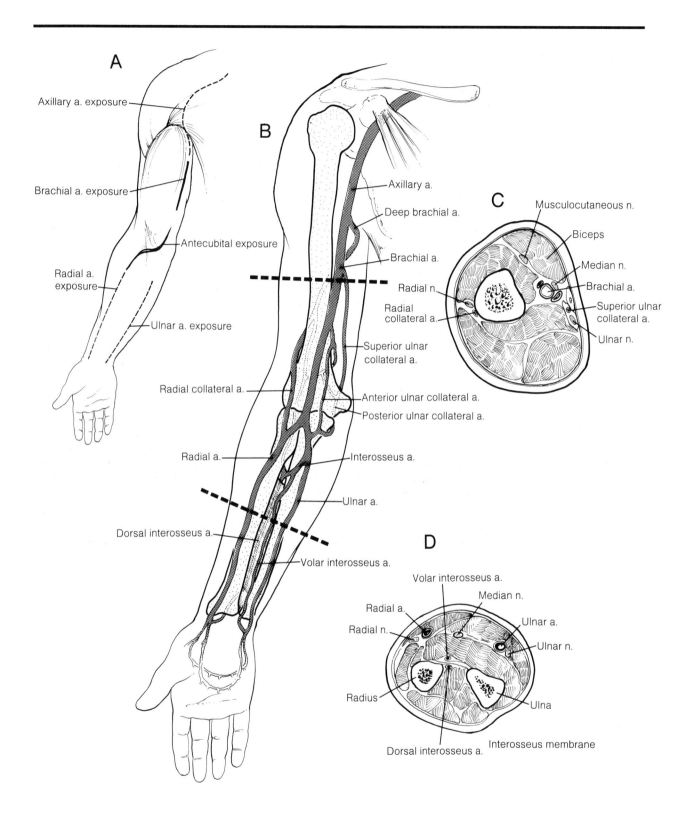

A

Axillary a. exposure

Brachial a. exposure

Antecubital exposure

Radial a. exposure

Ulnar a. exposure

B

Axillary a.

Deep brachial a.

Brachial a.

Superior ulnar collateral a.

Radial collateral a.

Anterior ulnar collateral a.

Posterior ulnar collateral a.

Radial a.

Interosseus a.

Ulnar a.

Dorsal interosseus a.

Volar interosseus a.

C

Musculocutaneous n.

Biceps

Median n.

Brachial a.

Superior ulnar collateral a.

Ulnar n.

Radial n.

Radial collateral a.

D

Volar interosseus a.

Median n.

Radial a.

Ulnar a.

Radial n.

Ulnar n.

Radius

Ulna

Dorsal interosseus a.

Interosseus membrane

Upper Extremity Arterial Exposure

Fig 11–2, A. The entire length of the axillary artery is exposed through an incision that originates parallel to the biceps muscle in the arm and takes a natural ''S'' across the axilla over the lateral margin of the pectoralis major in the delto-pectoral groove and parallels the clavicle. The arm is dropped into the operating field so that anterior traction on it will relax the pectoralis major for medial retraction and exposure of the underlying axillary contents. The pectoralis minor muscle may be mobilized or divided. The median nerve is in close proximity to the axillary artery. Alternatively, if only a short segment of the artery is required for exposure, the proximal portion may be exposed through a transverse incision on the anterior chest wall below the clavicle. The pectoralis muscle fibers are simply separated from the deltoid muscle in the delto-pectoral groove to gain access to the axillary artery on the chest wall.

B. Exposure of the brachial artery is through an incision parallel to the humerus placed in the groove between the biceps and triceps muscles. The brachial artery is found posterior to the biceps muscle with the median nerve overlying it.

C. Exposure of the brachial artery in the antecubital fossa requires retraction or division of the biceps aponeurosis. The median nerve is located anteromedial to the brachial artery. The brachial artery bifurcates to form the ulnar and radial arteries.

D. Exposure of the ulnar artery (or radial artery) in the forearm or at the wrist is via an incision parallel to its expected course. Muscle fibers and tendons are separated to isolate the artery.

E. Technique of arterial repair is dictated by extent of arterial injury. Clean laceration is usually repaired by mobilization of sufficient arterial length to allow end-to-end anastomosis. For larger arteries, simple continuous suture technique is used. For smaller arteries, triangulation suture technique is used. The space between triangulation sutures may be filled in with interrupted sutures, or continuous sutures may join the three stitches placed for orientation and exposure. When there has been a long segment of artery destroyed, interposition of a saphenous vein graft is the preferred treatment.

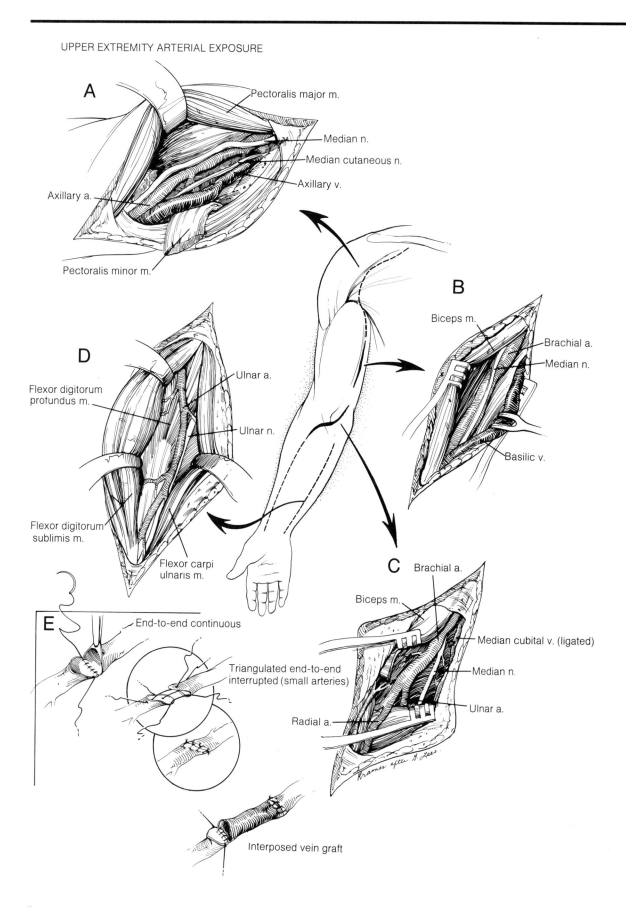

A
Pectoralis major m.
Median n.
Median cutaneous n.
Axillary a.
Axillary v.
Pectoralis minor m.

B
Biceps m.
Brachial a.
Median n.
Basilic v.

D
Ulnar a.
Flexor digitorum profundus m.
Ulnar n.
Flexor digitorum sublimis m.
Flexor carpi ulnaris m.

C
Brachial a.
Biceps m.
Median cubital v. (ligated)
Median n.
Ulnar a.
Radial a.

E
End-to-end continuous
Triangulated end-to-end interrupted (small arteries)
Interposed vein graft

Kramer after G. Lees

Aorto-femoral Artery Bypass

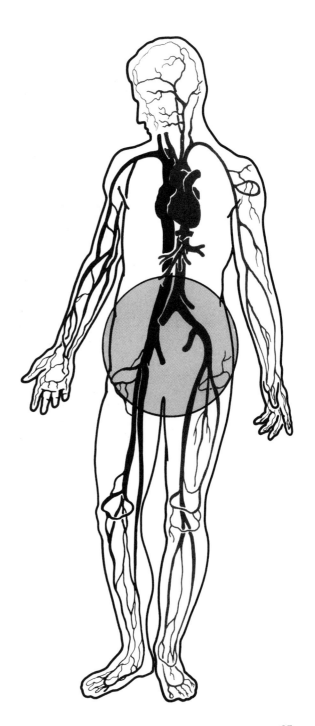

12

Fig 12–1. Bypass operations are performed to treat stenosis of the distal aorta and iliac arteries. The requirements for successful bypass are satisfactory inflow into the aorta below the renal arteries and satisfactory run-off arteries in the leg below the inguinal ligament. A midline incision is made that extends from xyphoid process to pubic ramus. Separate vertical incisions are made over the common femoral arteries beginning slightly above the inguinal ligament.

A. The common femoral arteries along with the superficial and profunda branches are mobilized and controlled with vessel loops.

B. The transverse portion of the colon and omentum are displaced outside the abdominal cavity superiorly onto moist laparotomy pads. The small intestine is either packed into the right lower quadrant or displaced outside the abdomen to the right in a Lahey bag. Packs are placed on the splenic flexure and sigmoid portions of the colon, and retracted by assistants or an adjustable retractor device fixed to the operating table. An incision is made in the peritoneum over the aorta just posterior to the fourth portion of the duodenum. The peritoneal incision extends from the Ligament of Treitz to the pelvic brim. A retroperitoneal tunnel is created by blunt dissection from the groin incisions to the pelvic brim along the anterior aspect of the iliac arteries. The ureters are mobilized anterior to the tunnel. Umbilical tape is drawn through the retroperitoneal tunnel for ease of location of the passageway later. The abdominal aorta is exposed from the level of the left renal vein to the inferior mesenteric artery. The proposed level of division of the aorta should be located in an area where the aortic wall is relatively free of atheromatous change. Heparin 100 to 200 units/kg is administered intravenously to increase the activated clotting time above 300 seconds prior to vascular occlusion.

C. The aorta is occluded just distal to the renal arteries and immediately proximal to the inferior mesenteric artery. The aorta is divided and a small portion excised. In patients with chronic occlusion of the infra-renal aorta, the renal arteries are controlled, occluded with vascular clamps, and the aorta clamped above the renal arteries. Thromboendarterectomy of the occluded aorta is performed using a Freer septum elevator. The obstructing material can usually be removed as a single intact plug. The renal artery orifices are inspected to be certain that no debris remains. The vessels are flushed with heparinized saline solution. The aortic clamp is moved to the infra-renal position and renal artery blood flow reestablished. Renal artery blood flow velocity is assessed with Doppler ultrasound using a sterile probe. A vascular clamp should never be applied to the aorta below the renal arteries if thrombus is present until the thrombus has been cleared as the debris may be squeezed superiorly into the renal arteries with catastrophic results.

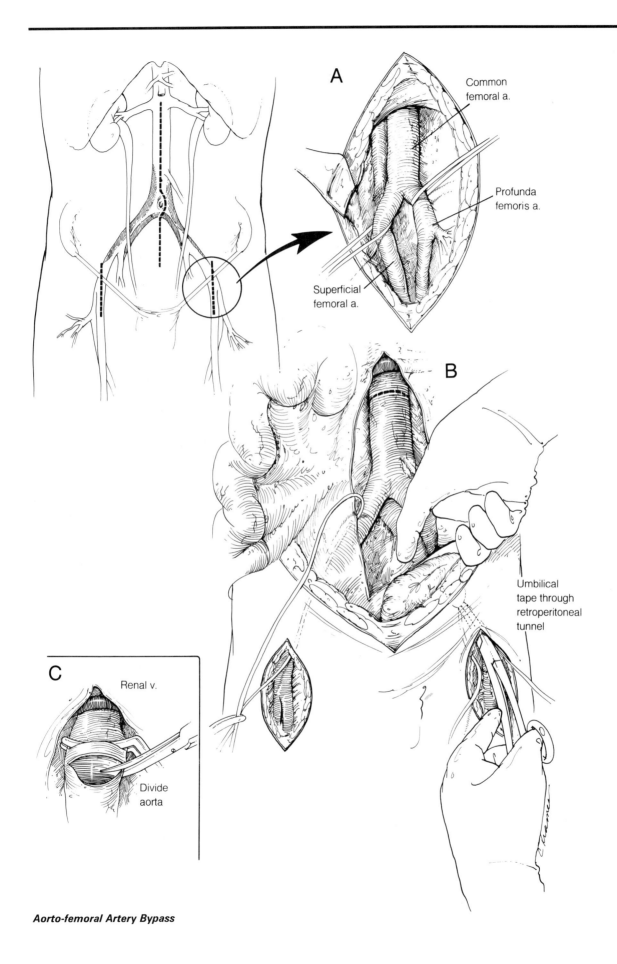

A

Common
femoral a.

Profunda
femoris a.

Superficial
femoral a.

B

Umbilical
tape through
retroperitoneal
tunnel

C

Renal v.

Divide
aorta

Fig 12–1, D. The distal end of the aorta is closed with 3/0 polypropylene suture. A continuous stitch is used, fashioned into a double row. The suture line is started posteriorly and continued to the anterior portion of the aorta. The suture may be continued as the second row back to the original point and secured or the opposite end of the suture used for the second row.

E. A vertically placed aortic clamp may be used to reduce dissection required posterior to the aorta, but the exposure of the posterior wall of the aorta is not as good as with an aortic clamp which closes the aorta from the side.

F. A Dacron prosthetic graft is selected that approximates the diameter of the aorta. A 16- to 18-mm graft will be chosen in most cases. Double velour knit Dacron sealed with heated (autoclave) albumin is the preferred material. The bifurcated graft is fashioned to provide a short length above the limbs. A 1.5- to 2.0-cm piece of the graft is cut and placed over the graft as a cuff to protect the proximal anastomosis. To facilitate placement of the posterior row sutures, the graft is held apart from the aorta as the suture loops are placed using a 3/0 double-armed polypropylene suture. The suture line is started outside the graft so that the needle will pass from the lumen of the aorta and through the adventitia to avoid the risk of elevating atheromatous plaques from the intimal surface. The suture line is started on the side of the aorta at a point away from the surgeon so that the suture line proceeds toward the surgeon. The graft is drawn into position by traction on the two free ends of the suture. With the graft approximating the aorta, the posterior row of sutures can be inspected. The suture line is continued to the right until most of the right lateral portion of the anastomosis is finished. Once the anterior portion of the aorta is approached, it is best to hold this suture and use the opposite end of the suture for the remainder of the stitches. The anastomosis is completed by taking the left limb of the suture around the aorta anteriorly.

G. An alternative end-to-side anastomosis of the graft to the aorta is only employed when the aorta is very small with complex anatomy requiring multiple vessel implantation into the graft or when there is total occlusion of the iliac vessels so that retroperfusion of the iliac, sacral, and lumbar arteries is impossible. A side occlusion clamp is used to isolate the anterior aspect of the infra-renal aorta. A vertical incision is made into the aorta. The bifurcated graft is beveled. Several stitches of 3/0 polypropylene are placed at the heel of the graft and through the distal end of the aortotomy prior to approximating the graft to the aorta.

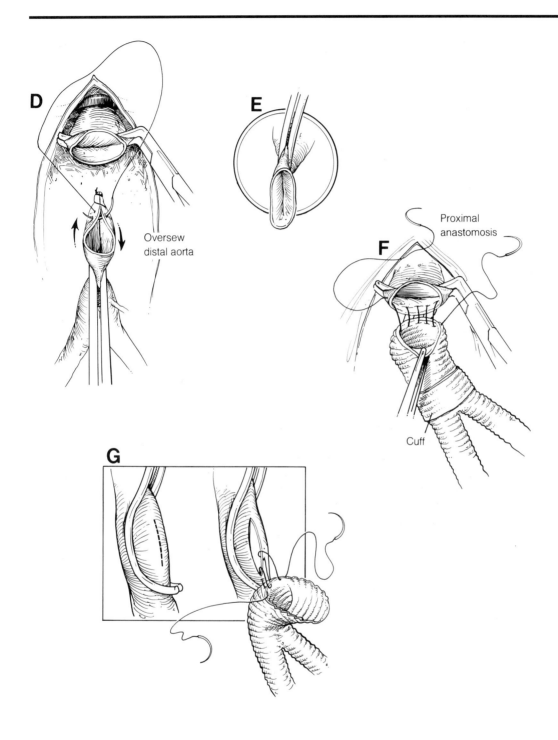

D

Oversew
distal aorta

E

F

Proximal
anastomosis

Cuff

G

Fig 12–1, H. Following completion of the proximal anastomosis, the aortic vascular clamp is opened while the graft is occluded to check the integrity of the anastomosis. The proximal aortic suture line may be covered with the short graft sleeve constructed from a portion of the unused proximal aortic graft. This is particularly important if the aorta required endarterectomy due to calcified plaques or chronic total aortic occlusion. One distal graft limb corresponding to the easiest distal anastomosis is pulled through previously formed retroperitoneal tunnels into the groins using a long aortic aneurysm clamp. The distal oversewn aorta should be placed exactly in the aortic graft bifurcation with the left graft limb usually placed beneath the inferior mesenteric artery. An incision is made in the femoral artery. If there is disease in the profunda femoris artery, the incision is extended onto the profunda femoris artery to its first bifurcation or beyond all occlusive disease. The graft limb is fashioned to the appropriate length by removing the excess graft and cutting the distal end into a bevel.

I. To facilitate placement of the initial sutures, the graft is held apart from the femoral artery. The end-to-side anastomosis is constructed with a continuous 4/0 or 5/0 polypropylene suture by placement of five suture loops between the heel of the graft and the proximal end of the arteriotomy.

J. The graft is drawn into position by traction on the free ends of the suture. The suture ends will hold the arteriotomy open by traction.

K. The anastomosis is continued along the right side of the arteriotomy around the distal apex. Suture loops may be left slightly loose until the apex is passed in order to better visualize the lumen of the artery. The anastomosis is completed along the left margin of the arteriotomy using the opposite end of the suture or simply by continuing with the original needle depending on individual circumstance and preference.

A soft jaw vascular clamp (Fogarty) is placed to occlude the origin of the graft limb which has been anastomosed to the femoral artery. The aortic clamp is briefly released to flush out the aorta via the unanastomosed limb of the graft. The soft jaw clamp is then moved to occlude the unanastomosed limb of the graft at its origin. The aortic clamp is gradually opened to establish flow to the lower extremity through the completed limb of the graft. The unanastomosed limb of the graft is cleared of any blood or clot by a suction tip passed inside the limb of the graft. This graft limb is then passed through the preformed tunnel into the groin incision where the femoral artery anastomosis is completed.

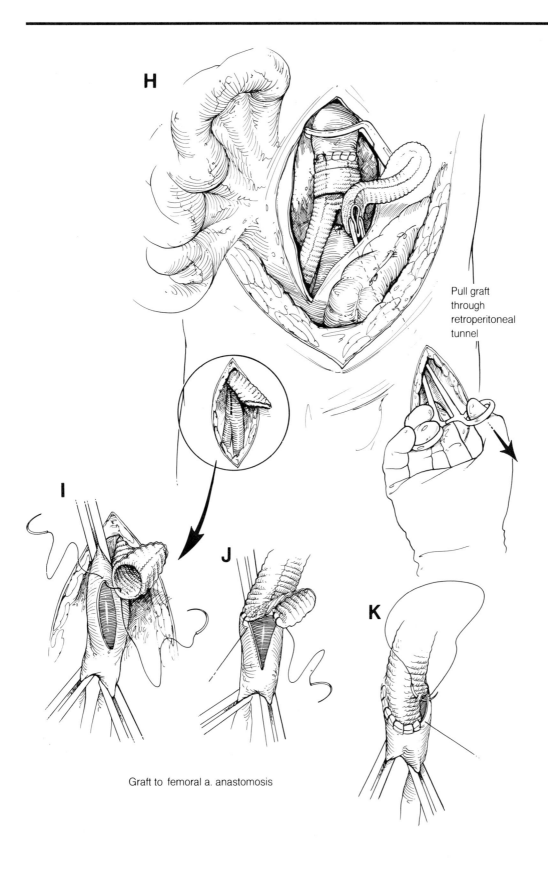

H

Pull graft through retroperitoneal tunnel

I

J

K

Graft to femoral a. anastomosis

Fig 12–1, L. Following completion of all anastomoses, blood flow is restored by removal of occlusive vascular clamps. Heparin effect is completely reversed with intravenous protamine to a baseline or normal activated clotting time. A Doppler velocity probe is used to assess the flow characteristics at the distal anastomosis and beyond as well as adequacy of inferior mesenteric artery blood flow. If necessary, the inferior mesenteric artery is replanted into the aortic graft.

The cuff is pulled around the proximal anastomosis to reinforce the repair and to guard against formation of false aneurysm which is thought to be a significant factor in late aorto-duodenal fistula formation. The completed repair should be isolated in the retroperitoneum by approximating the peritoneum in front of it. In some cases, a segment of omentum may be placed between the graft and the duodenum. Orderly replacement of the intestine and accurate closure of the abdominal wall are important details for uncomplicated recovery.

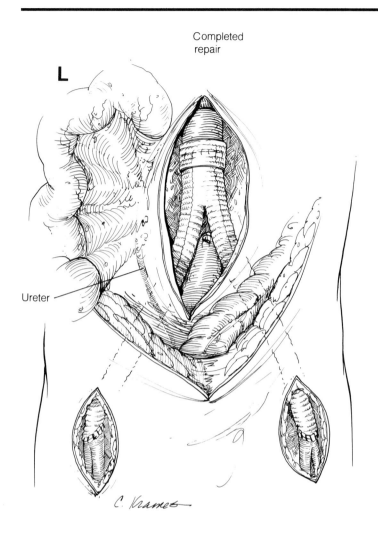

Completed
repair

L

Ureter

C. Kramer

Aorto-iliac
Endarterectomy

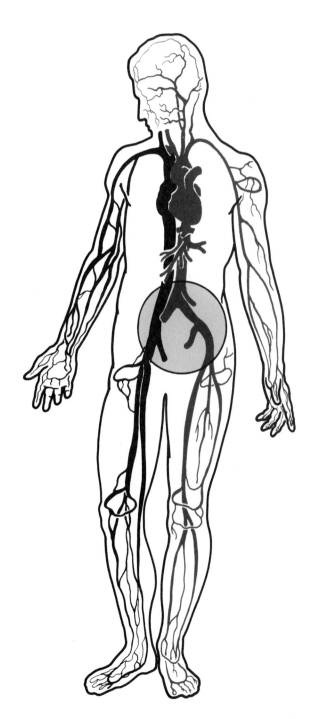

13

Fig 13–1. Aorto-iliac obstructive disease may be treated by endarterectomy technique in selected cases. The disease should be limited to the distal aorta and proximal iliac arteries. While more extensive disease can be treated with the endarterectomy extending into the femoral arteries, it is usually best to restrict this operation to more localized disease and use bypass operations for revascularization extending to the groin. Endarterectomy operations are usually done in younger patients because the procedure may be more time-consuming than bypass operations, and more extensive dissection of the aorto-iliac arterial segment is required. Because of the greater mobilization of the aortic bifurcation that is required, there is a greater tendency to disrupt the sacral neural plexus that courses through the aortic bifurcation as well as sympathetic innervation resulting in retrograde ejaculation in males. Nevertheless, this operation has the advantage that only autogenous blood vessels are used in the reconstruction and the only foreign material that will be utilized is the suture material to close the arteriotomies.

A midline incision extending from the xyphoid process of the sternum to the pubis is made. The abdominal contents are explored and a careful inspection and palpation of the arteries is done. Endarterectomy is considered if the atherosclerotic process ends in the common iliac arterial segment or in some cases where the disease extends on the posterior wall exclusively into the internal iliac arterial segment. The external iliac arteries should be normal to palpation and confirmed patent by preoperative arteriography. The transverse colon is placed onto moist laparotomy packs on the chest wall above the incision, and the small intestine is placed in a Lahey bowel bag and retracted to the right outside the abdomen. The peritoneum is incised over the aorta extending from the left renal vein to the iliac artery bifurcation on the right. An adjustable ring retractor that attaches to the operating table fixes the exposure and enhances the procedure.

A. The aorta distal to the cross point of the left renal vein is exposed. The aortic bifurcation is completely mobilized. The common iliac arteries are freed from the iliac veins that lie posterior to the arteries. The ureters are identified and retracted out of the operating field. Thorough mobilization of the arteries to be treated by endarterectomy is essential to the success of the operation. The internal iliac arteries should be freed up and controlled along with the proximal portion of the external iliac arteries.

B. The aorto-iliac arterial segment is isolated by vascular clamps placed on the distal aorta and on the internal and external iliac arteries. Longitudinal incisions are made at the aortic bifurcation and in the iliac arteries extending slightly into the external iliac segment so that the iliac bifurcation and the take-off of the internal iliac artery may be clearly exposed. Alternatively, two long arteriotomies may be made extending from the distal aorta all the way through the common iliac segment for direct exposure of the disease process. The advantage of the former approach is that less arterial incision will have to be closed at the expense of having a "blind" segment from which the disease must be removed. The advantage of the latter approach is obviously exposure for more accurate removal of the atherosclerotic plaque at the expense of a tedious closure of a long arteriotomy.

C. The atherosclerotic plaque is dissected away from the aortic adventitia by establishing a plane in the media layer that adequately removes the disease process. A Freer septum elevator is the best instrument for this job.

D. The atherosclerotic plaque is divided at the proximal end of the arteriotomy. With a little care, the plaque may be divided so that the plaque proximally remains tightly attached to the aortic wall. Sharp scissors may be used to remove any unwanted plaque so that the proximal edge is finished nicely.

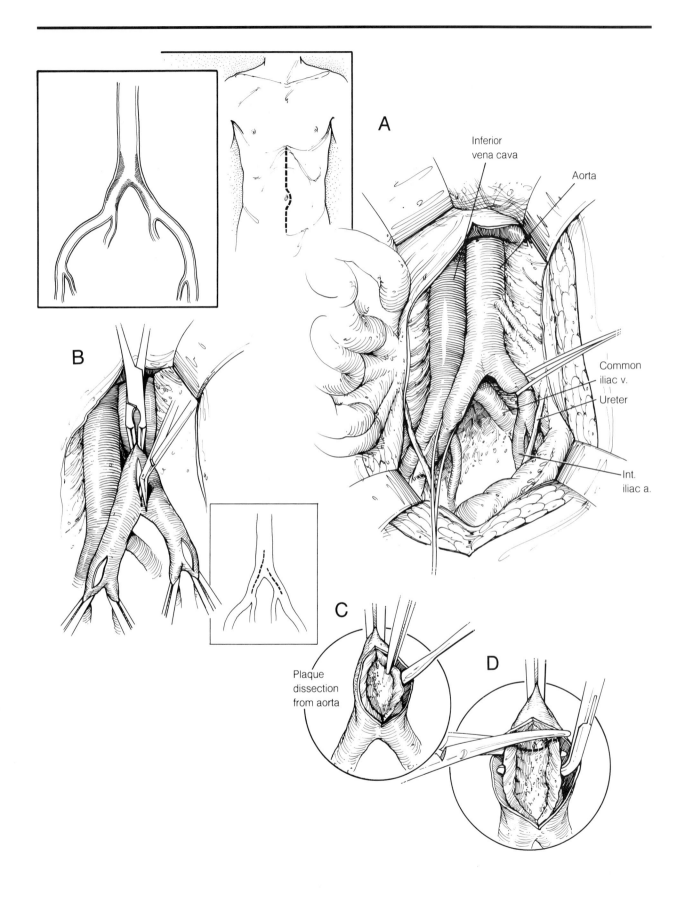

A

Inferior
vena cava

Aorta

Common
iliac v.

Ureter

Int.
iliac a.

B

C

Plaque
dissection
from aorta

D

Fig 13–1, E. The atherosclerotic plaque is separated from the arterial wall in the common iliac artery. The dissection is started proximally from the aorta into the iliac artery using the Freer septum elevator. The distal endpoint of the atherosclerotic plaque is established at the distal arteriotomy. The plaque is separated circumferentially and carefully tapered at the external iliac artery. Usually the bulk of the disease will tail off posteriorly into the internal iliac artery in properly selected cases. In some cases, it may be necessary to divide the atherosclerotic plaque at the external iliac artery. When this is done, care should be taken to assure that the remaining intima distally is tightly adherent to the arterial wall by using sharp scissors to cut the plaque against the artery. Where required, tacking stitches may be used, but it is better to actually end the plaque dissection by taper or accurate division than to depend on a few sutures to prevent intimal flap elevation.

F. The plaque is totally separated from the common iliac segment. The technique involves grasping the artery with the fingers of one hand while inserting a 35-degree DeBakey peripheral vascular clamp with the other hand. The fingers are used to compress the plaque and artery to the clamp inside the vessel and effect the separation of the plaque with the fingers rather than using a probing or tearing action with the clamp or other endarterectomy device. If "blind" endarterectomy is difficult and the plaque does not separate readily, the arteriotomy should be extended through the entire common iliac segment so that the plaque may be directly exposed for accurate dissection.

G. When bilateral endarterectomy is performed, it is best to divide the plaque at the aortic bifurcation and perform the endarterectomy of the common iliac segments separately. Following removal of the plaque, the iliac artery is thoroughly irrigated with saline solution containing heparin. A fine mesh gauze strip may also be drawn through this segment to assure that all atherosclerotic debris is removed. The artery should feel smooth and thin after completion of endarterectomy.

H. The repair is completed by closure of the arteriotomies by continuous stitches using 5/0 polypropylene suture. The alternative technique that utilizes long arteriotomies over the entire common iliac artery will require some time to effect closure.

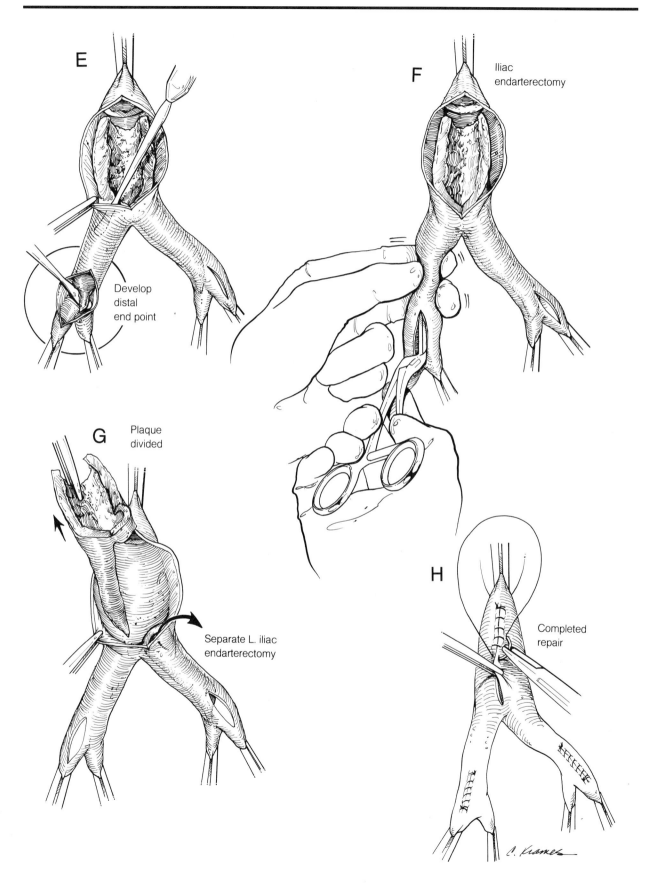

E

Develop distal end point

F

Iliac endarterectomy

G

Plaque divided

Separate L. iliac endarterectomy

H

Completed repair

C. Kramer

Extra-anatomic Bypass

14

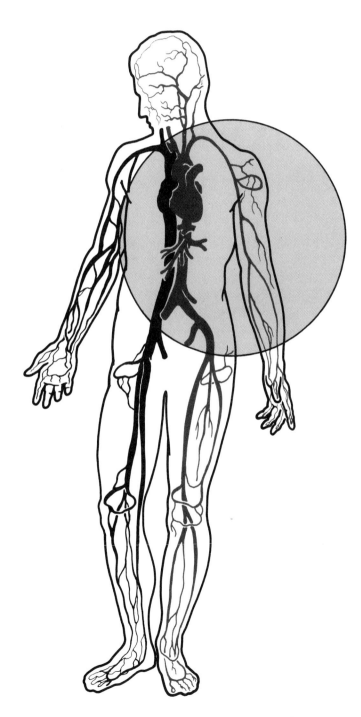

Femoral–Femoral Artery Bypass

Fig 14–1. Direct approach to an arterial lesion may not be desirable in some patients with arterial obstruction. Patients with reduced functional reserve due to cardiac or pulmonary insufficiency may not tolerate celiotomy or thoracotomy. Infection, prior radiation therapy, or multiple operative procedures may preclude operative approach to a particular anatomic site. In these patients, revascularization procedures may be accomplished more judiciously using some pathway that is apart from the usual anatomic location. Extra-anatomic bypass procedures are utilized in these cases.

An arterial lesion that is well-treated by extra-anatomic bypass is occlusion of the iliac artery in a patient where the opposite iliac artery carries blood flow unimpeded to the femoral artery. This lesion may be treated without entering the peritoneal cavity by bringing in flow from the unaffected femoral artery to the opposite affected femoral artery. The incisions for the procedure are placed in each groin over the common femoral arteries.

A. A subcutaneous tunnel is created between the groin incisions just above the pubic bone after completely freeing up each of the common femoral arteries.

B. A longitudinal arteriotomy is made in the common femoral artery on the affected side. A single vascular clamp may be used to isolate the arteriotomy site or individual clamps may be placed on the common femoral artery and its branches depending on operator preference.

C. An end-to-side anastomosis of a tubular prosthetic graft to the common femoral artery is constructed. If the superficial femoral artery is occluded or profunda femoris artery stenosis exists, a profundaplasty should be performed using the graft. The arteriotomy is extended onto the profunda femoris artery to its major bifurcation and the anastomosis of the graft made over the length of arterial incision. Polytetrafluoroethylene (PTFE-Goretex) tubular graft material is preferred at present although Dacron prostheses are quite acceptable. Graft size is usually 8–10 mm in diameter.

D. Sponge forceps or a DeBakey aneurysm clamp is passed through the subcutaneous tunnel and the graft pulled through. Attention is given to avoiding twist of the graft.

E. An end-to-side anastomosis of the graft to the inflow common femoral artery is constructed using 4/0 or 5/0 polypropylene suture material. The completed graft will thus have a curved course that has no known deleterious effects.

The completed bypass brings blood to the affected femoral artery from the opposite femoral artery via a bypass graft coursing through the subcutaneous tissues of the abdominal wall above the pubis. In younger, sexually active patients, it may be preferable to route the graft behind the rectus abdominus muscles via the retropubic space of Retzius so it is not vulnerable to compression.

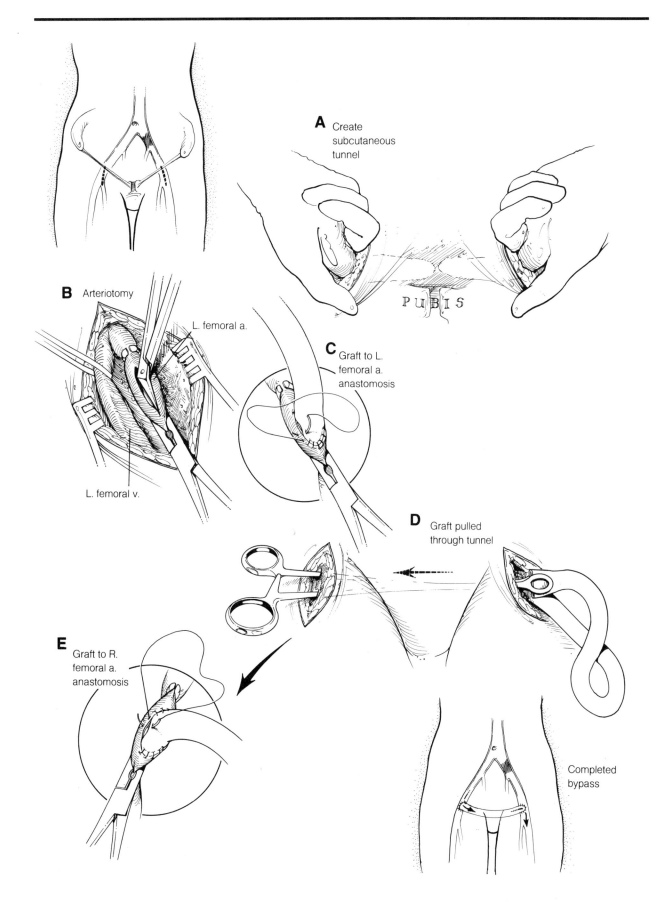

A Create subcutaneous tunnel

PUBIS

B Arteriotomy

L. femoral a.

L. femoral v.

C Graft to L. femoral a. anastomosis

D Graft pulled through tunnel

E Graft to R. femoral a. anastomosis

Completed bypass

Axillary-Femoral Artery Bypass

Fig 14–2. Revascularization of a limb when there is occlusion of the iliac artery and some disease of the opposite iliac artery, which renders it inadequate to supply blood flow to both extremities, is accomplished with bypass from the ipsilateral axillary artery.

Skin incisions are made below the clavicle and in the groin over the common femoral artery on the affected side. A small counter incision near the costal margin in the mid-axillary line is usually required to bring the bypass graft between the two primary incisions. The arm is prepared into the operating field so that it can be positioned to relieve tension on the pectoralis major muscle for optimal exposure to the axillary artery.

A. The pectoralis major muscle fibers are separated to expose the pectoralis minor muscle. The pectoralis minor is divided at its tendon.

B. The axillary artery is mobilized and dissected free of the axillary vein and brachial plexus.

C. A single curved vascular clamp is used to isolate a portion of the axillary artery. A longitudinal arteriotomy is made. It should be placed as close as possible to the chest wall to prevent movement with arm motion. An end-to-side anastomosis of a polytetrafluoroethylene (PTFE-Goretex) tubular prosthesis to the axillary artery is constructed by continuous stitch of 5/0 polypropylene suture. Five suture loops are placed at the "heel" of the beveled vascular prosthesis to the distal end of the arteriotomy prior to approximating the graft to the artery. Diameter of the prosthesis is usually 10 mm.

D. The proximal anastomosis is completed by bringing the continuous suture line around the "toe" of the graft.

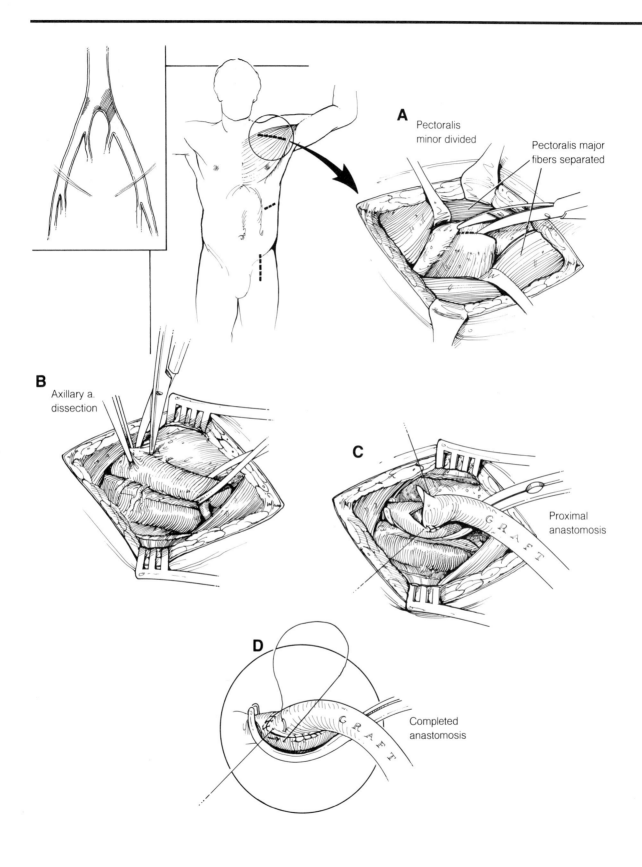

A Pectoralis minor divided

Pectoralis major fibers separated

B Axillary a. dissection

C Proximal anastomosis

D Completed anastomosis

Fig 14–2, E. A subcutaneous tunnel is created from the axilla to a counter incision near the costal margin. The distance is too great and the angles of the body are such that creating a tunnel from axilla to groin without counter incision is not practical. The graft is attached to the tunneler device and pulled through to the counter incision.

F. A subcutaneous tunnel is created from the groin to the counter incision. The graft is attached to the tunneler and graft pulled through the tunnel to the groin. Attention is given to avoiding twist of the graft under the skin.

G. An end-to-side anastomosis of the beveled graft to an arteriotomy in the common femoral artery is constructed using continuous stitches of 5/0 polypropylene suture material. Length of graft should be exact so that no kink is possible and no downward tension placed on the axillary artery.

H. The completed bypass brings input from the ipsilateral axillary artery to the common femoral artery. In almost all cases, a femoro-femoral graft anastomosis is constructed, which clearly improves the patency rate of this otherwise thrombosis prone graft. The incisions are closed using absorbable suture in the subcutaneous tissue to completely cover the graft and in the subcuticular layer of the dermis to approximate the skin edges.

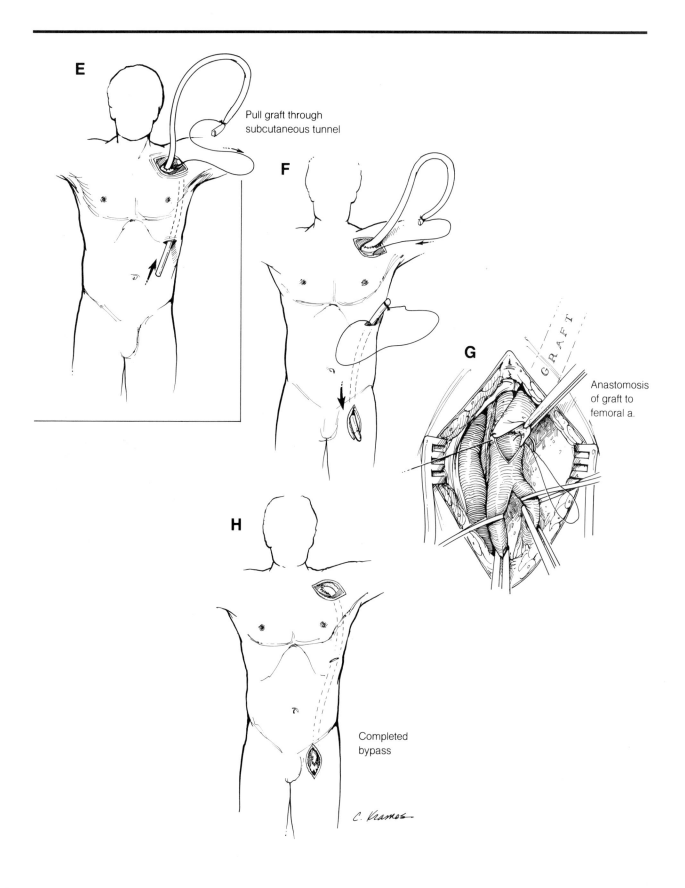

E

Pull graft through
subcutaneous tunnel

F

G

Anastomosis
of graft to
femoral a.

H

Completed
bypass

C. Krames

Axillary-Bilateral Femoral Artery Bypass

Fig 14–3. Total occlusion of the distal aorta may be relieved with bypass graft from the axillary artery to both femoral arteries in the groin. This graft reconstruction is most often used to revascularize the lower extremities following removal of an infected aorto-iliac graft. However, this outflow pathway from the upper compartment may be compromised in cross-sectional area.

A. Incisions are placed as described for axillary-femoral artery bypass and in the contralateral groin over the common femoral artery. The proximal anastomosis of a 10-mm polytetrafluoroethylene (PTFE-Goretex) graft to the axillary artery is constructed and the bypass graft pulled through a subcutaneous tunnel to the ipsilateral groin incision. Care is taken to course the graft in the midaxillary line as it crosses the rib cage to prevent acute angulation at the junction of ribs and the abdominal muscles.

B. Part of the end of the graft is removed to form a bypass to the opposite groin, or a second piece of slightly smaller (8-mm) graft is used. An end-to-side anastomosis of the two grafts is constructed using a running stitch of fine polypropylene suture. When PTFE graft is used, this anastomosis must be carefully constructed because needle-hole bleeding can be aggravating.

C. The primary graft is shortened and beveled to approximate the common femoral artery. An end-to-side anastomosis of graft to an arteriotomy in the common femoral artery is constructed using continuous stitches of 4/0 or 5/0 polypropylene suture.

D. The bypass is completed by creating a subcutaneous tunnel between the groin incisions as for femoral-femoral artery bypass and bringing the side-arm graft to the contralateral common femoral artery by end-to-side anastomosis.

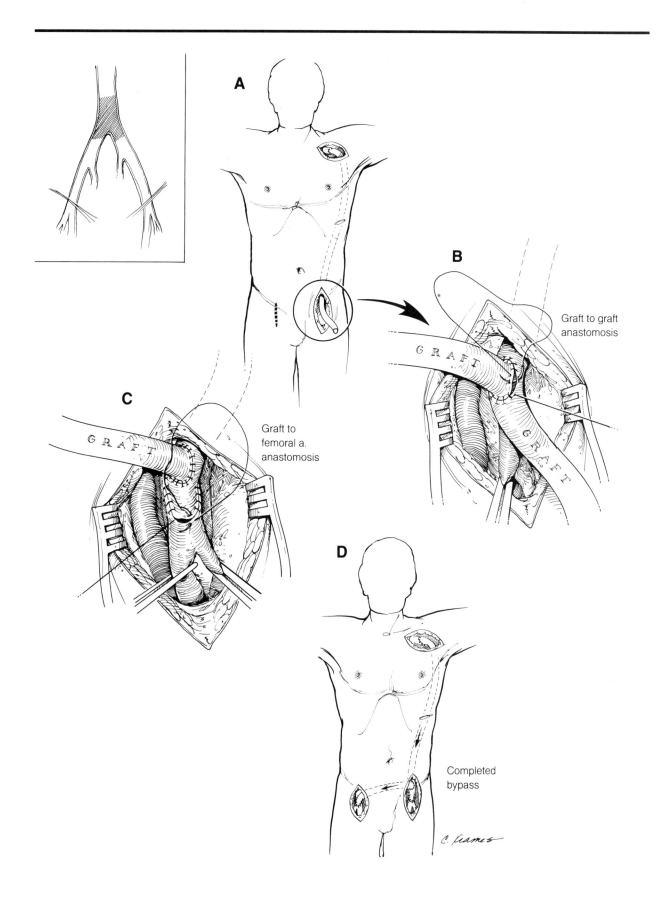

A

B

Graft to graft
anastomosis

C

Graft to
femoral a.
anastomosis

D

Completed
bypass

C. Reames

Ascending Aorta-Abdominal Aorta Bypass

Fig 14–4. Complex recurrent coarctation of the thoracic aorta, infection of thoracic aortic prosthetic grafts, and coarctation of the proximal abdominal aorta may be treated with bypass graft from the ascending aorta to the abdominal aorta distal to the obstruction.

A. A midline incision is made from the suprasternal notch to the umbilicus. The thymus is separated in the midline. The pericardium is opened at the upper portion to expose the ascending aorta. The peritoneum is opened with the incision extending a short distance into the diaphragm in the midline. Retraction sutures are placed in the pericardial sac. The left lobe of the liver is mobilized by dividing ligamentous attachments to the diaphragm and retracted to the right. The supraceliac portion of the abdominal aorta is mobilized. This portion of the aorta is located between the aortic crura of the diaphragm. The muscle fibers of the diaphragm must be mobilized and retracted or divided to obtain enough length on the aorta above the celiac artery. The aorta is separated from the vena cava on the right and the sides of the aorta freed up enough to apply a side-biting vascular clamp. The aorta is usually totally occluded by application of this clamp. The clamp should optimally be only partially occlusive of the aorta, but as a practical matter, it is better to achieve isolation of sufficient aorta so that the edges of an arteriotomy will be easy to separate than to worry about partial occlusion of the aorta to maintain blood flow distally.

B. An end-to-side anastomosis of a tubular Dacron prosthesis to the aorta is constructed. The graft is 16–20 mm in diameter depending on size of the patient and the ascending and abdominal aorta. The graft is knit double velour crimped Dacron that has been prepared by saturation with concentrated serum albumin and heated in the autoclave. The graft is cut without bevel and the arteriotomy made precisely to length. This anastomosis is deep in the abdominal cavity and exposure compressed by surrounding liver, diaphragm, and celiac axis. The anastomosis is completely constructed with graft held apart from the aorta. Once the graft and aorta are approximated, exposure is difficult because the graft fills the area. Continuous stitches of 3/0–4/0 polypropylene suture is used. Five suture loops are placed between graft and one end of the arteriotomy. The initial and final stitch of the five are placed near the midpoint of the arteriotomy on each side.

C. A second suture is used to place the five suture loops between graft and the other end of the arteriotomy. Thus, the needles on each end of the two sutures will come out of the middle of the graft on one side and out of the aorta on the other side. The suture loops are pulled up as the graft is approximated to the aorta. The ends of the sutures are joined by knot to secure the anastomosis.

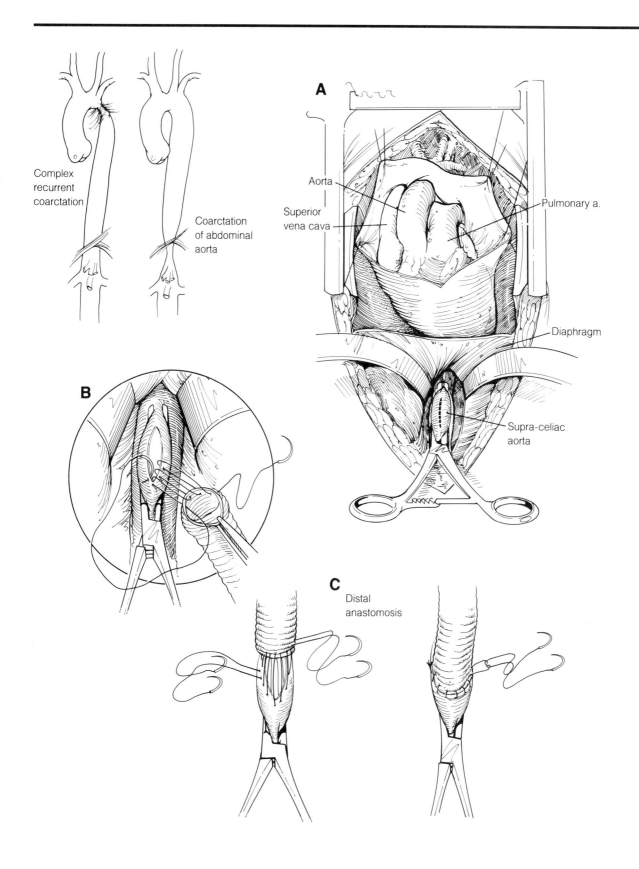

Complex
recurrent
coarctation

Coarctation
of abdominal
aorta

A

Aorta

Superior
vena cava

Pulmonary a.

Diaphragm

Supra-celiac
aorta

B

C Distal
anastomosis

Fig 14–4. The graft is occluded near the abdominal aortic anastomosis with a soft-jaw clamp (angled Fogarty) so that the aortic occlusion clamp may be removed, the anastomosis tested for hemostasis, and blood flow restored to the distal aorta. A side-occlusion clamp (Lambert-Kay) is applied to the ascending aorta, making sure that the degree of obstruction of the aorta will be tolerated. An arteriotomy is made in the ascending aorta in the portion isolated by the vascular clamp. The bypass graft takes a course from the abdominal aorta, below the diaphragm, to the mediastinum in front of the pericardium. The graft is shortened by bevel to appropriate length to approximate the ascending aorta.

E. An end-to-side anastomosis of the graft to the ascending aorta is constructed with continuous stitches of 3/0 polypropylene suture. The initial five suture loops are placed between ''heel'' of graft and proximal end of the arteriotomy prior to approximating the graft to the aorta.

The completed bypass graft from ascending aorta to supraceliac abdominal aorta effectively restores blood flow and avoids approach to complex pathology in the upper portion of the descending thoracic aorta. For pathology involving the supraceliac portion of the abdominal aorta such as coarctation of the abdominal aorta, it may be preferable to bypass to the infrarenal portion of the abdominal aorta. However, the latter procedure exposes more of the abdominal viscera to the graft with the potential for erosion. The graft may be tunneled beneath the peritoneum around the abdominal wall if deemed desirable.

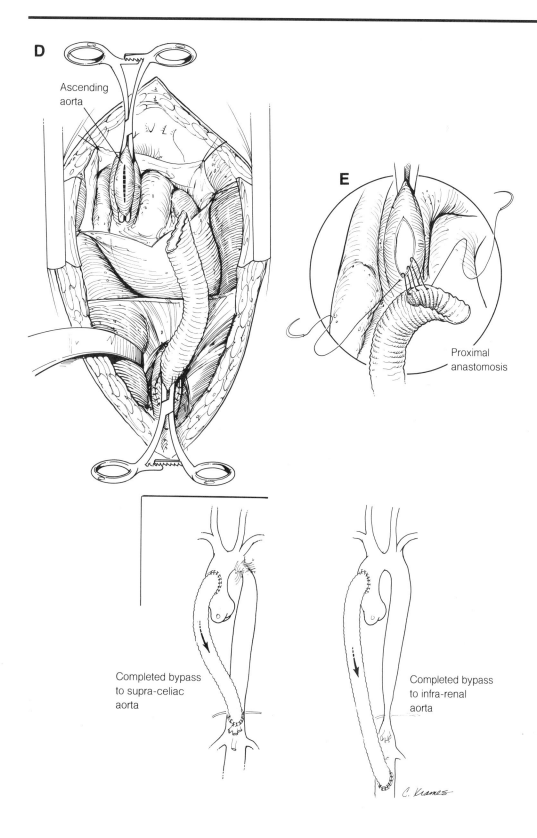

D

Ascending aorta

E

Proximal anastomosis

Completed bypass to supra-celiac aorta

Completed bypass to infra-renal aorta

C. Krames

15

Profundaplasty

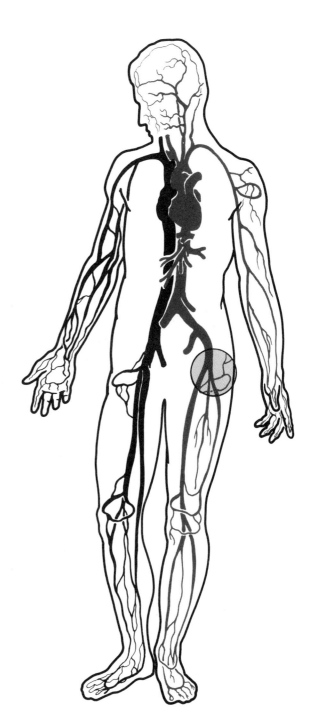

Fig 15–1. The profunda femoris or deep femoral artery provides extremely important blood supply to the leg. Atherosclerotic disease, which limits blood flow through this artery, will often place the limb in danger of distal necrosis when it is commonly associated with proximal occlusion of the superficial femoral artery. Restoration of good blood flow to the deep femoral system will usually save the limb even when there is other significant limb vascular occlusion. Profundaplasty is usually combined with an inflow procedure (aorto-femoral or femoro-femoral bypass). If inflow is good, it is combined with an outflow operation (femoro-popliteal or femoro-distal artery bypass). It is rarely used alone in current practice.

A. The most common method of profunda femoris reconstruction (profundaplasty) is in combination with aorto-femoral bypass graft procedures. The incision in the common femoral artery is extended onto the profunda femoris artery.

B. The arteriotomy is carefully extended beyond the atherosclerotic disease process. The disease in the proximal artery is left undisturbed to avoid disruption of the normal intima of the profunda artery distally. The dissection of the artery and the arteriotomy is always taken to the first branch point or beyond, where the disease usually ends. The profundaplasty must be carried to the first major bifurcation so that the cross-sectional area is increased, thus relieving the relative stenosis of the profunda femoris when associated with superficial femoral artery occlusion. The profunda femoris dissection may be extended for a considerable distance into the leg and the arteriotomy extended the length of the dissection, but the complexities of reconstruction are magnified with greater length required to complete the repair.

C. The tubular Dacron prosthesis, which is usually part of an aorto-femoral revascularization procedure, is used to open out the stenosed profunda artery. The graft is beveled to appropriate length to completely cover the arteriotomy. The heel of the graft is attached to the proximal end of the arteriotomy by placing five continuous stitches while the graft is held apart from the artery.

D. Stitches are placed around the distal end of the arteriotomy with precision so that the graft actually widens the artery. Sutures must be placed with gentleness and precision as the profunda femoris is a thin, fragile, and unforgiving artery. The suture loops are left slightly loose until the apex is completed so that the lumen may be accurately visualized.

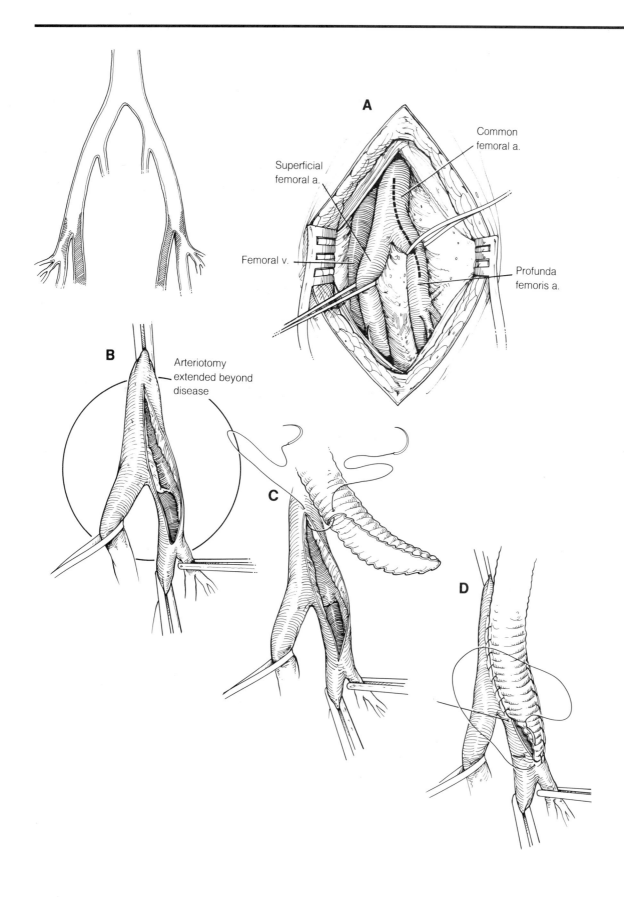

A

Common femoral a.

Superficial femoral a.

Femoral v.

Profunda femoris a.

B

Arteriotomy extended beyond disease

C

D

Fig 15–2, A. Profundaplasty may be performed by thromboendarterectomy technique, provided that the atherosclerotic process extends only a short distance into the profunda femoris artery. After appropriate dissection and control of the branches of the common femoral artery, an incision is made into the common femoral artery near the takeoff of the profunda and extended onto the profunda to its first major bifurcation.

B. The thromboendarterectomy dissection is started in the media-adventitia plane in the common femoral artery, mobilizing the plaque away from the adventitial layer.

C. The plaque is separated from the back wall of the common femoral artery so that circumferential dissection is completed. The plaque is divided at the proximal end.

D. The dissection is taken a short distance into the superficial femoral artery, which is usually occluded. The plaque is divided in the superficial femoral artery so that only the extension of the plaque into the profunda femoris remains.

E. The Freer septum elevator is gently passed into the profunda femoris to separate the plaque from the artery. The distal tip must be separated without raising a flap of the intima. Extreme care and patience should be used at this point of the dissection. The plaque is separated from the profunda femoris artery and extracted. It is often helpful to release the occlusion clamp before removing the plaque.

F. The distal intima should be visualized to be sure that it is solidly attached. If there is any question about the distal end point, the intima is tacked down with 6/0 polypropylene suture.

G. The arteriotomy is closed with a patch; if the profundaplasty is performed as part of a bypass graft procedure, the prosthetic graft is used to close the arteriotomy in the usual fashion.

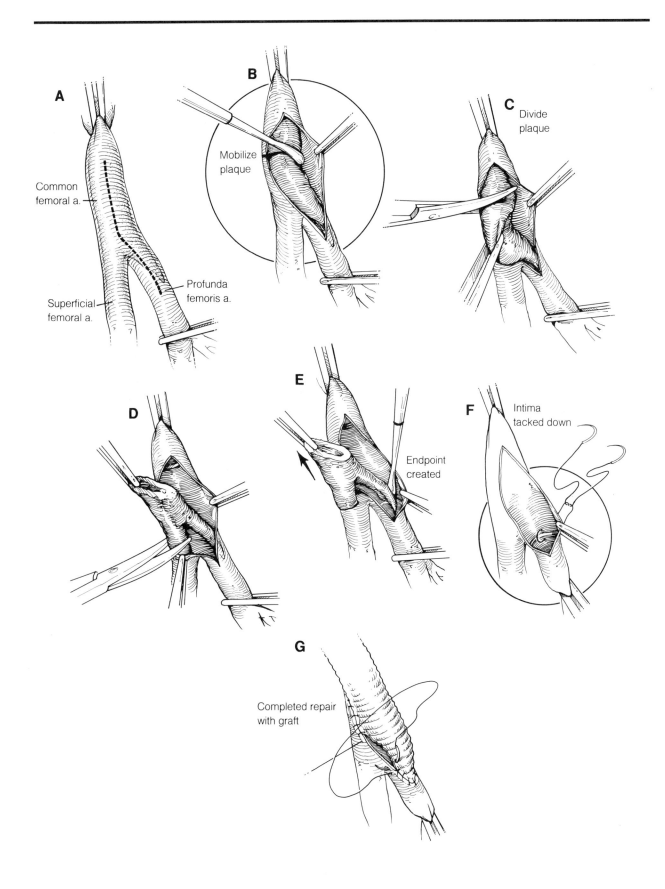

A

Common femoral a.

Superficial femoral a.

Profunda femoris a.

B

Mobilize plaque

C

Divide plaque

D

E

Endpoint created

F

Intima tacked down

G

Completed repair with graft

Fig 15–3, A.   When the disease process in the femoral artery involves total occlusion of the superficial femoral artery and the plaque extends well into the profunda femoris artery such that the artery is thin, small, and branching where it becomes more normal, it may be desirable to reconstruct the profunda femoris artery with the superficial femoral artery after endarterectomy so that soft autogenous tissue is used at the distal tip of the profunda femoris arteriotomy. The superficial femoral artery is ligated and divided at a point approximately the length of the proposed incision of the profunda femoris artery. The incision of the femoral artery is extended into the profunda femoris artery past the disease process, at least to its first major bifurcation and into the superficial femoral artery to the point of division.

B.   A thromboendarterectomy of the common femoral, profunda femoris, and proximal superficial femoral artery is performed using the Freer septum elevator.

C.   The superficial femoral artery is used to widen out the profunda femoris artery. A continuous stitch of 5/0 polypropylene is started at the junction of the superficial femoral artery with the profunda femoris artery. The edge of the superficial femoral artery is joined to the edge of the arteriotomy of the profunda femoris artery.

D.   The suture line is continued to the apex of the arteriotomy of the profunda artery. The stitches at the apex are left loose until the apex is passed so that the stitches may be placed with precision. The suture line is continued joining the opposite side of the superficial femoral artery to the lateral edge of the arteriotomy of the profunda femoris artery, thereby enlarging the proximal profunda artery by the circumference of the superficial femoral artery.

E.   Alternatively, the suture line may be closed up to the common femoral artery, leaving a portion open for attachment of a prosthetic graft. This allows the stiff, non-compliant prosthetic material to be attached to a very wide part of the artery rather than to the thin and perhaps small lumen of the profunda artery distally. The heel of the graft is attached by several loose loops prior to approximating the graft to the artery.

The anastomosis is completed in the usual fashion by continuous stitches using 5/0 polypropylene suture.

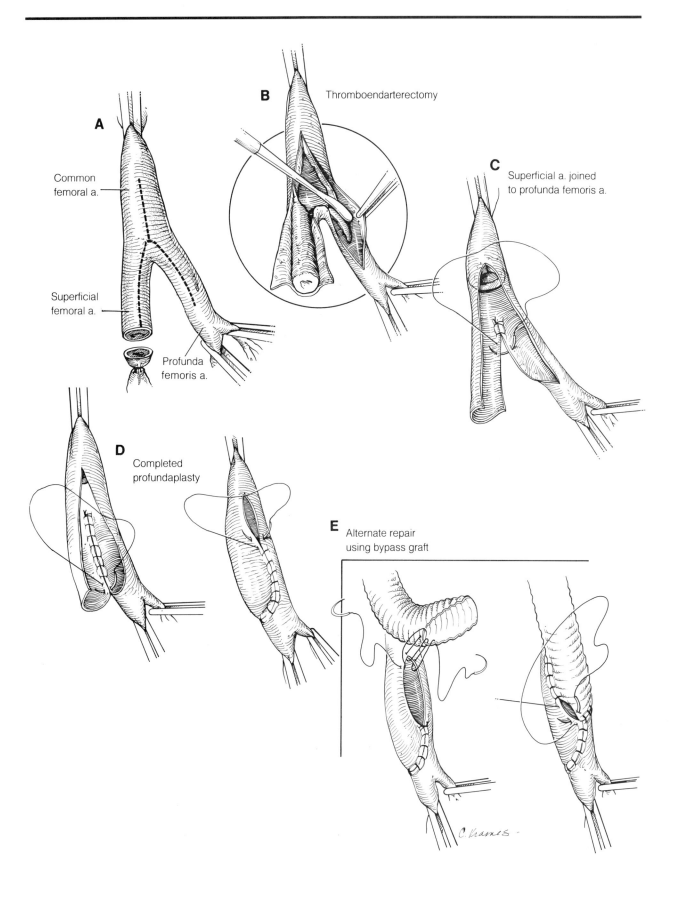

A

Common
femoral a.

Superficial
femoral a.

Profunda
femoris a.

B Thromboendarterectomy

C Superficial a. joined
to profunda femoris a.

D Completed
profundaplasty

E Alternate repair
using bypass graft

C. Kranes-

Complications of Aorto-ileo-femoral Artery Procedures

16

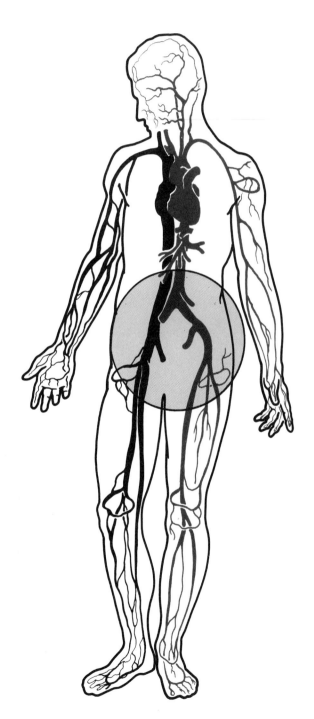

Reoperation for Late Occlusion in Single Limb Aorto-femoral Bypass

Fig 16–1. Thrombosis of one limb of a bifurcated aorto-femoral prosthesis can often be relieved without the necessity of replacement of the graft. Occlusion of a single limb of an aortofemoral graft with patency of the other limb usually occurs when there is outflow obstruction in the vessels to which the limb of the graft is attached. Typically, the affected limb of the graft is anastomosed to the common femoral artery and there is occlusion of the superficial femoral artery and stenosis of the origin of the profunda femoris artery.

A. The operative approach is through the original groin incision on the affected side. The graft and the branches of the femoral artery are mobilized and controlled. The superficial femoral artery is usually occluded and the profunda femoris artery is usually stenosed at its origin. The graft is opened longitudinally near the anastomosis to inspect the orifice of the profunda femoris artery from within the common femoral artery.

B. The graft is divided proximal to the anastomosis. The profunda femoris is opened by incision through its orifice. The arteriotomy is extended beyond the area of stenosis in the profunda artery to the first bifurcation point or beyond.

C. An embolectomy catheter is passed proximally through the graft into the aorta. The balloon is inflated and the thrombus in the graft extracted as the catheter is withdrawn. Recent thrombus is easy to remove and the procedure can be successful in thrombosed grafts as late as two weeks after graft closure. Care must be taken to prevent embolization of the opposite graft limb. Passing the embolectomy catheter only part way up the occluded limb with simultaneous temporary occlusion of the opposite graft limb with external manual compression in the groin may be helpful.

D. A new segment of graft is anastomosed to the end of the original graft to extend the length of the graft. The graft is beveled appropriately and with sufficient length to cover the arteriotomy beyond the area of profunda femoris artery stenosis. The initial five suture loops are placed in the heel of the graft prior to approximating graft to artery in end-to-side fashion.

E. The anastomosis is completed by continuous suture technique around the toe of the new segment of graft.

Several alternative approaches are available. The entire limb of a thrombosed graft may be replaced when the thrombus cannot be effectively removed by embolectomy catheter. A femoral artery to femoral artery bypass graft may be constructed to bring blood flow from the side with graft limb patency to the affected side. The entire bifurcated aorto-femoral graft can be replaced.

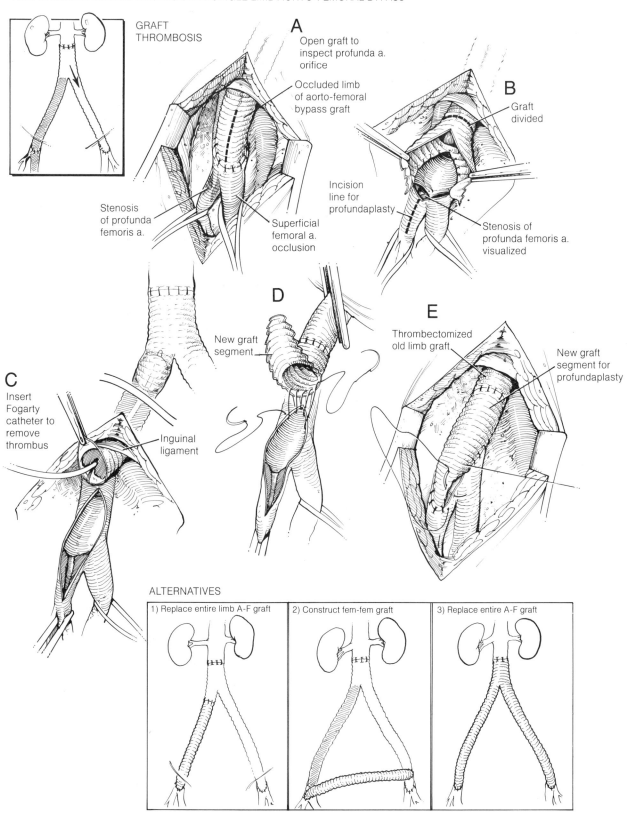

GRAFT THROMBOSIS

A
Open graft to inspect profunda a. orifice

Occluded limb of aorto-femoral bypass graft

B
Graft divided

Incision line for profundaplasty

Stenosis of profunda femoris a.

Superficial femoral a. occlusion

Stenosis of profunda femoris a. visualized

C
Insert Fogarty catheter to remove thrombus

Inguinal ligament

D
New graft segment

E
Thrombectomized old limb graft

New graft segment for profundaplasty

ALTERNATIVES

1) Replace entire limb A-F graft

2) Construct fem-fem graft

3) Replace entire A-F graft

Complications of Aorto-ileo-femoral Artery Procedures

Repair of Femoral Anastomotic False Aneurysm

Fig 16–2. False aneurysm occurring at the anastomosis of a prosthetic graft to the femoral artery is usually the result of dehiscence of the anastomosis. Nevertheless, routine cultures for bacteria and fungi should be performed to exclude the presence of infection.

A. The original groin incision used to make the anastomosis is reopened and the affected area exposed. The graft can usually be identified and controlled. It is more difficult to identify and control the femoral artery and its branches so that no attempt is made to do so.

B. After systemic administration of heparin, the prosthetic graft is occluded by vascular clamp. The false aneurysm is incised and back bleeding controlled by inflating balloon catheters within the lumen of the respective vessels. The superficial femoral artery is usually occluded from atherosclerotic disease. The graft is divided proximal to the anastomosis. The anastomosis is taken down and the graft removed from the femoral artery.

C. A new segment of graft is anastomosed to the original graft in end-to-end fashion. The new graft segment is shortened and beveled appropriately to approximate the arteriotomy in the common femoral artery. An end-to-side anastomosis of graft to common femoral artery is constructed by continuous suture technique. The balloon occlusion catheters are removed prior to completion of the anastomosis.

D. The completed repair lies within the false aneurysm restoring blood flow to the leg.

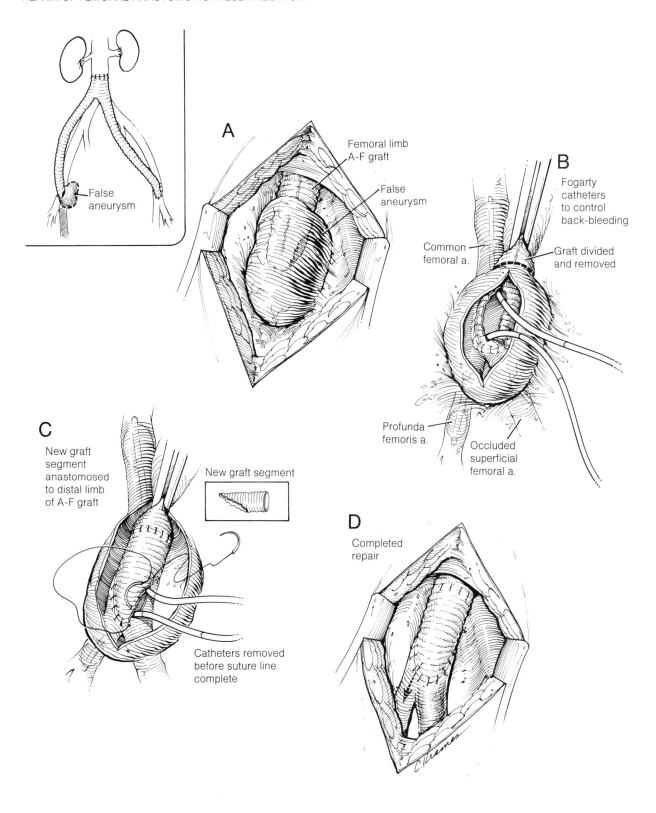

False aneurysm

A

Femoral limb
A-F graft

False
aneurysm

B

Fogarty
catheters
to control
back-bleeding

Common
femoral a.

Graft divided
and removed

Profunda
femoris a.

Occluded
superficial
femoral a.

C

New graft
segment
anastomosed
to distal limb
of A-F graft

New graft segment

Catheters removed
before suture line
complete

D

Completed
repair

Graft Infection of Groin

Bypass Through Obturator Foramen

Fig 16–3. Infection of the groin wound following aortobifemoral bypass graft should be treated aggressively when the prosthetic material becomes exposed and involved in the purulent process. The principles followed during reoperation are removal of the affected limb of the graft and restoration of limb blood flow through a tract separate from the original one. The previous midline abdominal incision is reopened or the affected limb of the bypass graft is approached through a new transverse lower abdominal incision and retroperitoneal dissection. The superficial femoral artery is approached through an incision on the medial aspect of the leg separate from the purulent process in the groin.

A. The affected limb of the bypass graft is exposed in an uninfected area in the retroperitoneum near its bifurcation. The graft is occluded and divided. The distal end is oversewn and the peritoneum closed over the old graft tract. A new graft tract is established from the retroperitoneum to the leg via the obturator foramen in the pelvis.

B. The anatomy of the lateral pelvic wall is presented to provide better understanding of the course of the new tract to the obturator foramen. The proximal end of the graft lies anterior to the common iliac artery near the sacral promontory at the pelvic brim. The distal end of the old graft is related to the external iliac artery and crosses into the groin anterior to the pubic ramus. The new graft tract will exit the pelvis into the leg posterior to the pubic ramus through the obturator foramen. The obturator internus muscle lines the lateral pelvic wall. The obturator nerve and artery course across the pelvic wall and exit to the leg through the antero-lateral aspect of the obturator foramen. The obturator foramen is covered by the peritoneum and a thick membrane that must be incised to allow passage of the graft to the leg.

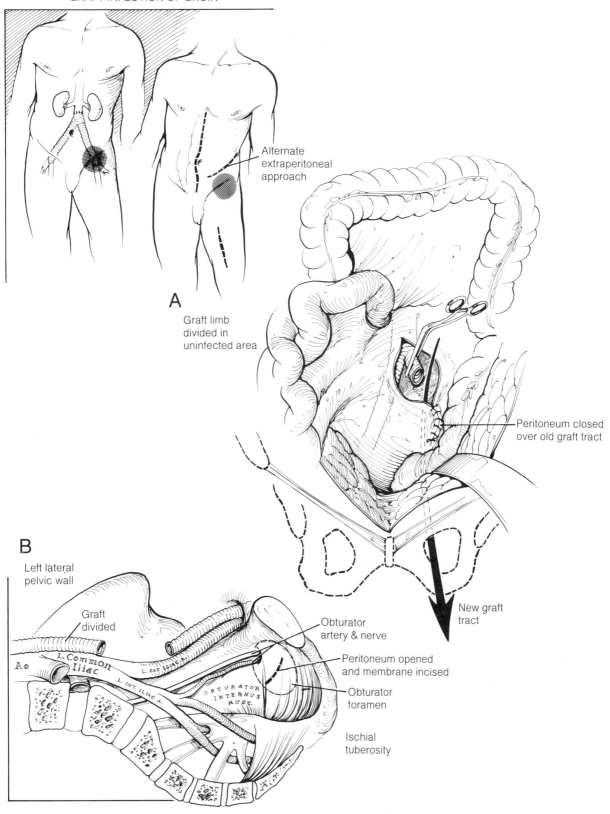

Alternate
extraperitoneal
approach

A

Graft limb
divided in
uninfected area

Peritoneum closed
over old graft tract

New graft
tract

B

Left lateral
pelvic wall

Graft
divided

Obturator
artery & nerve

Peritoneum opened
and membrane incised

Obturator
foramen

Ao.

L. Common
Iliac

L. EXT. ILIAC A.

L. INT. ILIAC A.

OBTURATOR
INTERNUS
MUSC.

Ischial
tuberosity

Fig 16–3, C. An incision on the medial aspect of the thigh is used to expose the superficial femoral artery. This incision should be placed well separated from the infected area in the groin. A tract in the retroperitoneum which leads to the obturator foramen is made by blunt dissection. An aneurysm clamp is used to create a tract from the incision on the medial aspect of the leg toward the obturator foramen. With the finger placed in the obturator foramen from above, the clamp is guided through the foramen medial to the obturator neurovascular bundle.

D. An end-to-end anastomosis of a new graft segment is made to the stump of the old affected limb of the bypass graft. The new graft limb is drawn across the retroperitoneum through the obturator foramen into the incision in the leg.

E. An end-to-side anastomosis of the new limb of the bypass graft to the superficial femoral artery is constructed. If the superficial femoral artery is occluded, the graft is placed to the profunda femoris artery or the proximal portion of the popliteal artery above the knee. The leg incision is closed to isolate the new graft. The purulent groin wound is opened as the final step of the procedure. The infected limb of the graft is pulled out of the graft tract and removed from the femoral artery. The femoral artery is repaired by closure with polypropylene suture.

F. The sartorius muscle is detached from its origin from the iliac crest. It is mobilized and rotated medially to cover the repair of the femoral artery. The muscle is attached to the inguinal ligament to maintain its position in covering the arterial repair. The subcutaneous tissue and skin are left open and the wound packed with acetic acid or betadine-soaked fine mesh gauze. The wound is allowed to heal by secondary intention.

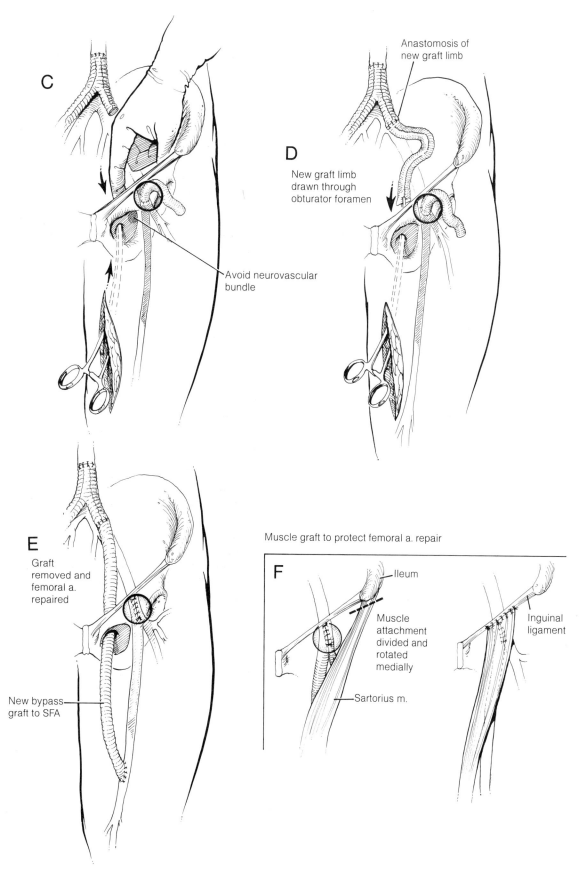

C

Avoid neurovascular bundle

D

Anastomosis of new graft limb

New graft limb drawn through obturator foramen

E

Graft removed and femoral a. repaired

New bypass graft to SFA

Muscle graft to protect femoral a. repair

F

Ileum

Muscle attachment divided and rotated medially

Sartorius m.

Inguinal ligament

Aorto-enteric Fistula

Fig 16–4. Fistula between the aorta and the third portion of the duodenum is a devastating complication of aortic surgery. There are two problems to be treated: (1) hemorrhage into the gastrointestinal tract resulting from direct communication of the aorta to the duodenum; and (2) sepsis resulting from communication of the duodenum with the blood stream. The aortic graft is always infected and must be removed.

A. The fistula between the aorta and duodenum is associated with false aneurysm of the anastomosis of aorta to the prosthetic graft. Less commonly, there is direct erosion of the prosthetic graft into the bowel without involvement of the suture line. Regardless of pathogenesis, the principles of management are the same.

B. Control of the aorta requires that the vascular clamp be placed initially proximal to the renal arteries. The area of the fistula is usually dense with inflammatory tissue, and approach to the aorta in the region of the false aneurysm may result in uncontrollable hemorrhage.

C. There is usually fistula from the duodenum to a false aneurysm leading to the proximal anastomosis of the aorta to prosthetic graft. The left renal vein is closely related to the inflammatory process, and it may be necessary to divide it in order to expose enough aorta below the renal arteries for control.

D. Whenever possible, the aortic occlusion clamp should be moved below the renal arteries. The graft is separated from the aorta. The duodenum is freed from the false aneurysm and the fistula closed in layers. Wide debridement of all involved tissues including the aorta is important to prevent dehiscence of the suture lines and recurrent fistula. The end of the aorta is closed by continuous horizontal mattress stitch and oversewn with continuous suture using 2/0 or 3/0 polypropylene.

E. The aortic closure is covered by a pedicle of omentum which is sutured to surrounding tissues to keep it in place. This maneuver also separates the duodenal closure from the aortic closure. The prosthetic graft is usually only loosely adherent and surrounded by purulent material. The entire graft is removed and the distal end of the arterial connection closed with polypropylene by oversewing the point of distal anastomosis. Gastrostomy with the tube passed into the proximal duodenum for drainage and jejunostomy for feeding are performed. Drains usually will be required in the bed of the infected graft if there is substantial purulent collection. The abdomen is completely closed. Restoration of lower extremity blood flow is by extra-anatomic bypass.

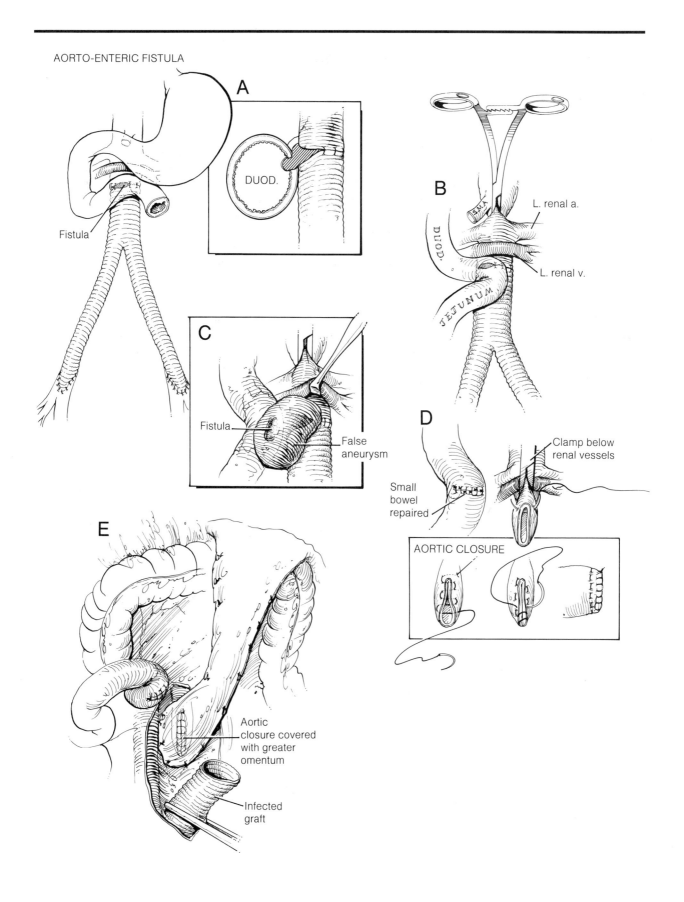

A

DUOD.

Fistula

B

SMA

DUOD.

JEJUNUM

L. renal a.

L. renal v.

C

Fistula

False
aneurysm

D

Small
bowel
repaired

Clamp below
renal vessels

AORTIC CLOSURE

E

Aortic
closure covered
with greater
omentum

Infected
graft

Extra-anatomic Bypass for Aorto-enteric Fistula

Reconstruction for Intra-abdominal Graft

Fig 16–5. When aorto-enteric fistula occurs with a prosthetic graft which is completely within the abdomen such as an aorto-bilateral iliac artery bypass, the graft is removed and the end of the aorta and the anastomotic points on the iliac arteries are oversewn. Extra-anatomic bypass is performed with blood flow to the lower extremities originating from an axillary artery. A unilateral bypass graft from axillary artery to common femoral artery is constructed using a vascular prosthesis. A second prosthetic limb is attached to the bypass graft and taken across the supra-pubic area to the opposite common femoral artery. Constructing an axillo-bifemoral graft has a better patency rate than bilateral axillo-femoral grafts.

Reconstruction for Graft to Femoral Arteries

When aorto-enteric fistula is associated with prosthetic graft to the common femoral arteries, the groin area is considered to be contaminated. Complete removal of the graft is performed and the points of anastomosis closed. Extra-anatomic bypass is through prosthetic grafts based on both axillary arteries and brought through subcutaneous tunnels placed as far lateral to the original incisions in the groin as possible. The bypass grafts are attached to the superficial femoral or profunda femoris arteries in an area well separated from the groin.

RECONSTRUCTION FOR INTRA-ABDOMINAL GRAFT

RECONSTRUCTION FOR GRAFT
TO FEMORAL ARTERIES

Femoro-popliteal Artery Bypass

17

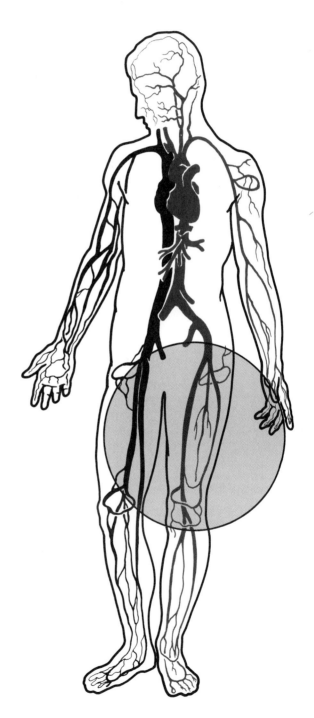

Anatomic Variations of the Popliteal Artery and Its Branches

Fig 17–1. Illustrated are four anatomic patterns of tibial and peroneal artery origin from the popliteal artery with cross-sectional anatomy at two levels below knee. Understanding these patterns is important in planning operation and for interpretation of arteriography.

Normal Popliteal Artery Configuration

A. The normal or most common pattern is for the popliteal artery to give rise to the anterior tibial artery immediately below the level of the knee. The anterior tibial artery penetrates the interosseous membrane between the tibia and fibula and courses distally along this membrane at the base of the anterior compartment. The popliteal artery continues as the tibio-peroneal trunk 4 or 5 cm before dividing into the posterior tibial artery and the peroneal artery which course distally behind the tibia in the deep compartment. As they progress distally, the posterior tibial artery becomes progressively more medial and finally reaches the ankle posterior to the medial malleolus. The peroneal artery courses distally beneath the fibula, finally terminating in branches to the antero-lateral aspect of the dorsum of the foot.

High Origin of the Anterior Tibial Artery

B. This anatomic variant is the same as the normal vascular arrangement except that the anterior tibial artery arises higher than normal at a level at or above the knee joint. In this situation, the tibioperoneal trunk bifurcates at a slightly higher level also.

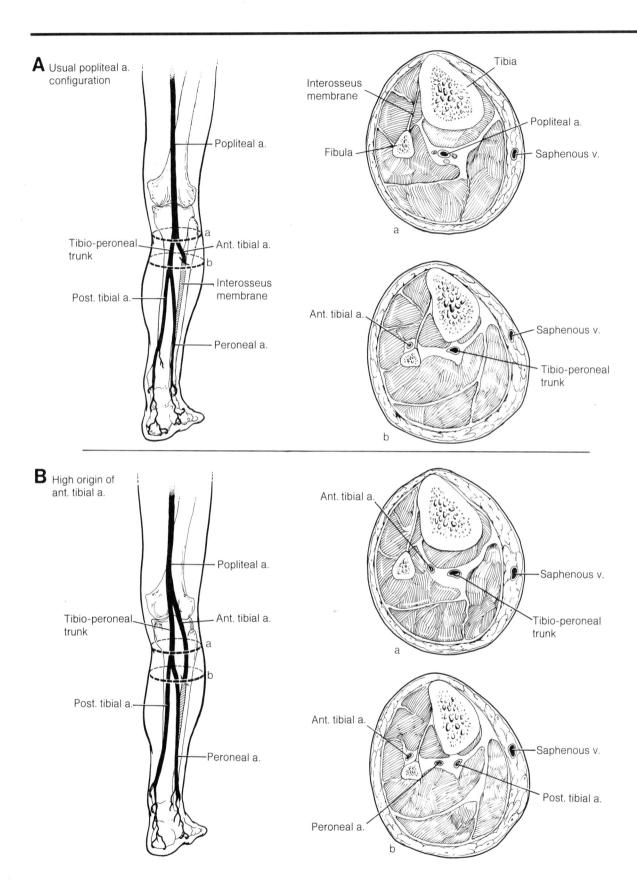

A Usual popliteal a. configuration

Popliteal a.

a

Tibio-peroneal trunk

Ant. tibial a.

b

Post. tibial a.

Interosseus membrane

Peroneal a.

Interosseus membrane

Tibia

Fibula

Popliteal a.

Saphenous v.

a

Ant. tibial a.

Saphenous v.

Tibio-peroneal trunk

b

B High origin of ant. tibial a.

Popliteal a.

Tibio-peroneal trunk

Ant. tibial a.

a

b

Post. tibial a.

Peroneal a.

Ant. tibial a.

Saphenous v.

Tibio-peroneal trunk

a

Ant. tibial a.

Saphenous v.

Post. tibial a.

Peroneal a.

b

Femoro-popliteal Artery Bypass

Anterior Tibial-Peroneal Trunk

Fig 17–1, C. This anatomic variant consists of high origin of the anterior tibial artery from the popliteal artery and origin of the peroneal artery from the anterior tibial artery immediately before it penetrates the interosseous membrane to enter the anterior compartment of the leg. The peroneal artery takes a normal course adjacent and deep to the fibula. The posterior tibial artery therefore originates higher than normal slightly below the knee and follows a normal course posterior to the tibia to the ankle.

Trifurcation of Popliteal Artery

D. This anatomic arrangement is uncommon and consists of a true trifurcation of the popliteal artery slightly below the knee. The artery divides simultaneously into three branches: anterior tibial, posterior tibial, and peroneal arteries. The three branch arteries follow the expected normal pathway to the ankle.

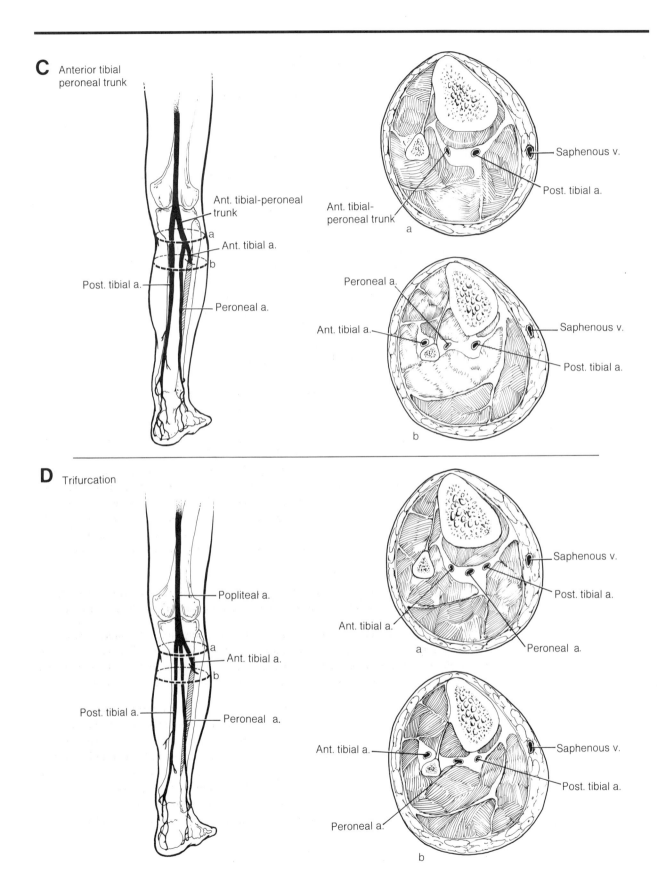

C Anterior tibial peroneal trunk

Ant. tibial-peroneal trunk

Ant. tibial a.

Post. tibial a.

Peroneal a.

Saphenous v.

Post. tibial a.

Ant. tibial-peroneal trunk

a

Peroneal a.

Ant. tibial a.

Saphenous v.

Post. tibial a.

b

D Trifurcation

Popliteal a.

Ant. tibial a.

Post. tibial a.

Peroneal a.

Saphenous v.

Post. tibial a.

Ant. tibial a.

Peroneal a.

a

Ant. tibial a.

Saphenous v.

Post. tibial a.

Peroneal a.

b

Femoro-popliteal Artery Bypass

Femoro-popliteal Artery Bypass, Reversed Saphenous Vein

Fig 17–2. The anatomic diagrams presented in this chapter to introduce and illustrate the pathology will follow the convention that arteries filled in solid (black) are patent and available for revascularization. This convention is followed for emphasis and clarity of illustration.

The patient who is a candidate for femoro-popliteal artery bypass has superficial femoral artery occlusion and a small or poorly developed profunda femoris artery. There are two methods to perform femoro-popliteal artery bypass using saphenous vein: (1) the traditional removal of the vein and bypass in the reversed position; and (2) bypass with vein in its natural position (in situ).

A. The patient is positioned supine with the abdomen from below the umbilicus and both legs to the ankle prepared into the operating field. The foot on the affected side is placed within a sterile plastic bag (Lahey), to permit visualization of it. The leg is flexed on a stack of towels or a rolled sheet. The incision to expose the saphenous vein is started in the groin 2 cm medial to the femoral artery pulse and 2 cm above the inguinal ligament. The incision is continued distally following the exact course of the saphenous vein. The skin and subcutaneous tissues are divided precisely vertical to the vein so that no flap is created. The vein is exposed sequentially and the skin incision extended as the course of the vein is known. The incision and exposure of the vein graft is continued for a distance below the medial condyle of the femur to a level approximating that estimated for arterial anastomosis. The vein is left in its bed while the popliteal artery is exposed through an incision in the deep fascia posterior to the saphenous vein. The popliteal space is entered and retractors placed for exposure. The popliteal artery is identified and separated from the popliteal vein and tibial nerve by sharp dissection. The artery is examined and findings correlated with the preoperative arteriography. The common femoral, superficial femoral, and profunda femoris arteries are exposed and controlled through the superior portion of the incision. Heparin is administered to achieve systemic anticoagulant effect. The saphenous vein is divided at its junction with the common femoral vein. It is progressively elevated from its bed while identifying the branches and dividing them after ligation with 4/0 silk against the vein graft and a hemoclip.

B. The vein graft is divided at the distal end of the incision. It is tied to a irrigating needle or cannula and gently distended and checked for security of closure of branches.

C. The popliteal artery is controlled proximally and distally with angled peripheral vascular clamps (DeBakey). A longitudinal arteriotomy is made. The saphenous vein graft is placed in reversed position, that is, with the end taken from the common femoral vein placed in the popliteal fossa. A 45 degree bevel is created at the end of the graft.

D. The anastomosis is constructed with 5/0 or 6/0 polypropylene and continuous suture technique. The initial five suture loops are placed between the heel of the graft and the proximal apex of the arteriotomy prior to approximating graft to artery. The suturing begins on the side away from the surgeon from the outside of the vein and continues from the inside of the artery. Lateral traction on both ends of the suture draws the heel of the graft into position against the artery. Side traction on the ends of the suture also help to separate the edges of the arteriotomy for better exposure. Suturing is continued in a clockwise direction until the apex of the arteriotomy is closed to the graft.

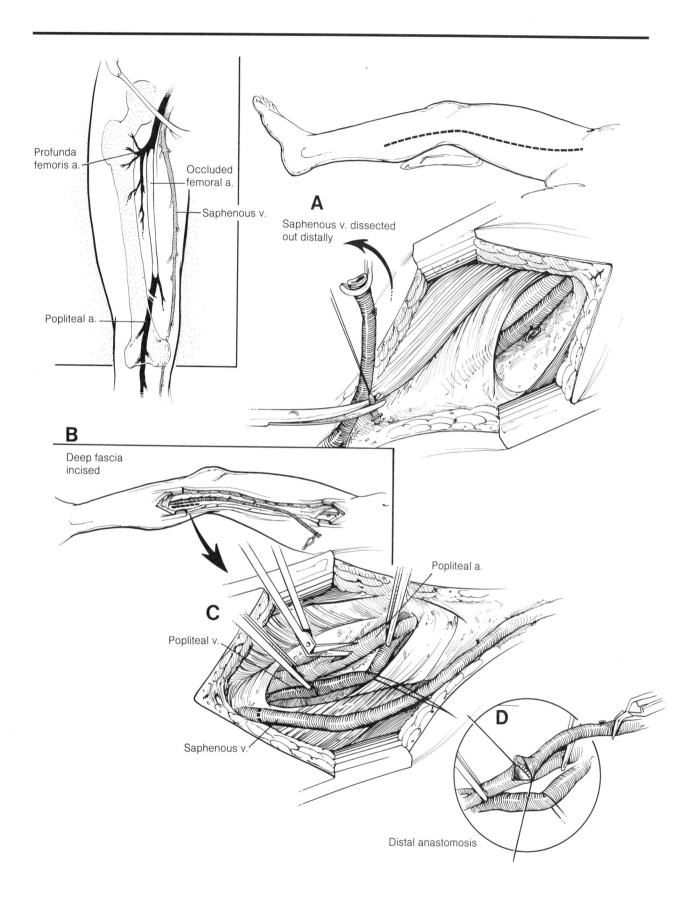

Profunda femoris a.

Occluded femoral a.

Saphenous v.

Popliteal a.

A

Saphenous v. dissected out distally

B

Deep fascia incised

C

Popliteal a.

Popliteal v.

Saphenous v.

D

Distal anastomosis

Fig 17–2, E. A tunneling device is passed from the groin to the popliteal fossa in a plane deep to the sartorius muscle. One hand is used to guide the tunneler, and the index finger of the other hand is placed in the popliteal fossa between the two heads of the gastrocnemius muscle. Proprioception will guide the tunneler to the popliteal space. The tunneler should not be passed through the medial or lateral heads of the gastrocnemius lest iatrogenic popliteal entrapment syndrome be induced. The saphenous vein graft is attached to the tunneler by the previously secured irrigating device. It is gently distended again to work out twisting of the graft. The tunneler is removed to the groin, pulling the vein graft through the leg into the incision above. The leg is straightened so that the required length of the vein graft may be accurately determined.

F. The common femoral, superficial femoral, and profunda femoris arteries are occluded with 35-degree angled peripheral vascular clamps (DeBakey). An arteriotomy is made in the common femoral artery opposite the origin of the profunda femoris artery. The profunda orifice is inspected for presence of stenosis from within the arteriotomy. The saphenous vein graft is shortened to appropriate length for anastomosis to the common femoral artery by dividing it at a 45-degree angle. The heel of the graft is cut back longitudinally to achieve enough length to cover the arteriotomy. An end-to-side anastomosis of the vein graft to the femoral arteriotomy is constructed using 5/0 or 6/0 polypropylene suture. Continuous suture technique is used. The initial five suture loops are placed at the heel of the graft and the distal apex of the arteriotomy beginning on the side away from the surgeon. The anastomosis is continued in clockwise fashion around the toe of the graft to complete the anastomosis. The vein graft is temporarily occluded while blood flow is restored to the leg through the profunda femoris artery. The graft is opened and blood flow through it assessed with Doppler ultrasound using a sterile probe. Blood flow in the popliteal artery distal to the bypass anastomosis is assessed similarly. A completion angiogram is performed.

G. The completed repair brings blood flow through the reversed saphenous vein bypass route to the popliteal artery beyond the area of obstruction of the artery. Hemostasis must be secure before closing the fascia, subcutaneous tissues, and skin in layers using absorbable polyglycolic acid suture material.

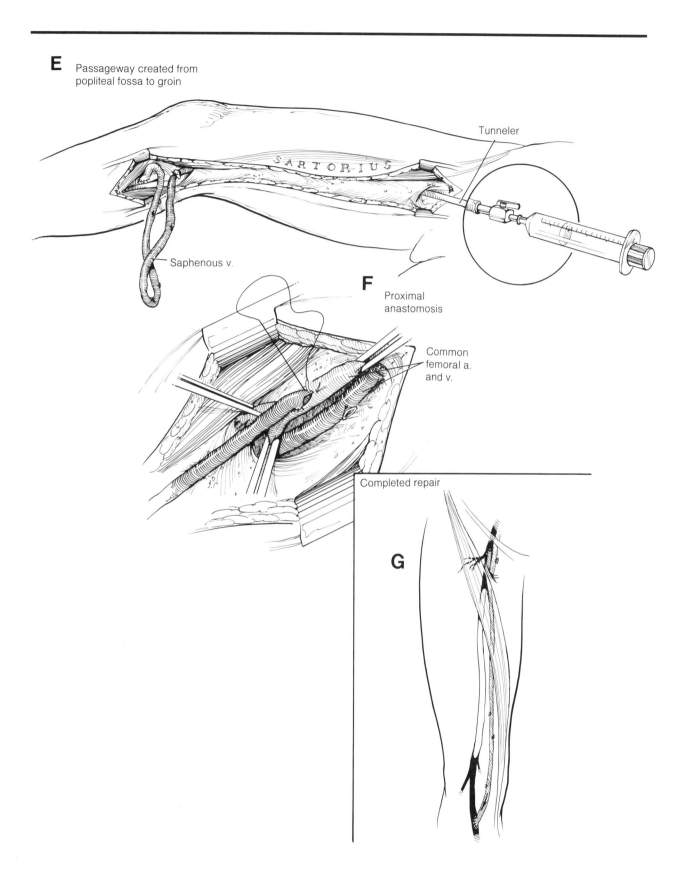

E Passageway created from popliteal fossa to groin

Tunneler

S A R T O R I U S

Saphenous v.

F Proximal anastomosis

Common femoral a. and v.

Completed repair

G

In Situ Saphenous Vein Graft

Fig 17–3. This operation is performed in exactly the same anatomic situation and for the same indications as the reversed saphenous vein bypass graft procedure. The advantages of the in situ technique are: (1) probable improved long-term patency (controversial); (2) better size match between artery and vein graft at both proximal and distal anastomoses; and (3) less possibility of twist or rotation of the vein graft during construction of the bypass. The disadvantages are: (1) superficial position of the graft in relation to the skin, especially near the knee so that skin necrosis or infection could be catastrophic; (2) the vein graft must be adequate in the leg affected by atherosclerotic occlusive disease; and (3) the valves in the vein graft must be destroyed with potential damage to intima with unknown late effects (probably not important).

The patient is positioned supine and prepared and draped from umbilicus to ankle on both sides. The affected leg is flexed over a stack of towels or a rolled sheet and the foot placed into a clear plastic bag (Lahey bag). A skin incision is made over the course of the saphenous vein.

A. The common femoral pulse is used as a guide for the skin incision which should be made 2 cm medial to it and started 2 cm above the inguinal ligament. The saphenous vein is carefully exposed by following it in its bed using scissors (Mayo curved) to separate the perivascular connective tissue and then dividing the subcutaneous tissue and skin precisely vertical to the vein to avoid creating a skin flap. The incision is continued to expose sufficient vein to reach the desired point of anastomosis. The branches of the vein are not disturbed at this point. The popliteal artery is exposed through an incision in the deep fascia posterior to the saphenous vein. The artery is freed from the accompanying vein and tibial nerve and controlled with vessel loops. It is inspected to be certain that it is satisfactory to accept the bypass graft.

B. The common femoral, superficial femoral, and profunda femoris arteries are isolated and controlled. The common femoral vein is identified and its junction with the saphenous vein exposed. Heparin is administered intravenously to achieve systemic anticoagulant effect. A curved vascular clamp (Cooley or Derra) is placed on the common femoral vein to isolate the saphenous vein junction. The saphenous vein is removed from the common femoral vein by excising it along with a small cuff of the femoral vein to increase the diameter and length of the graft origin. This also makes anastomosis of the vein graft to the femoral artery easier.

C. The common femoral vein is closed by continuous stitch of 5/0 polypropylene in a double row. Care must be taken not to create stenosis of the common femoral vein, and venous flow velocity should be evaluated in the vein by Doppler ultrasound after release of the occlusion clamp.

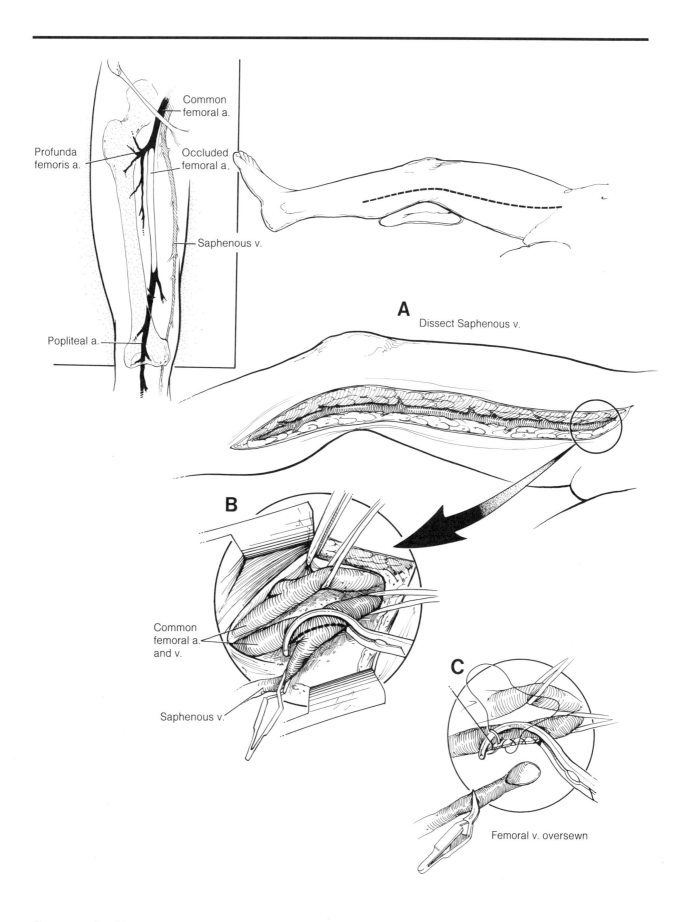

Common
femoral a.

Profunda
femoris a.

Occluded
femoral a.

Saphenous v.

Popliteal a.

A   Dissect Saphenous v.

B

Common
femoral a.
and v.

Saphenous v.

C

Femoral v. oversewn

Fig 17–3, D. The proximal saphenous vein is carefully straightened and held with forceps under slight tension so that valve microscissors (Karmody-Leather) can be safely introduced into the vein. One or two valves are cut and rendered incompetent. The first valve is immediately within the vein 0.5–1.0 cm from the end. The bicuspid venous valves are oriented such that the cusps close parallel to the skin. Thus, the microscissors are oriented so that the blades open and close perpendicular to the skin surface, assuring that the anterior blade will enter the anterior cusp and the posterior blade will enter the posterior cusp. Closing the blades divides the valve cusps in the mid-portion, rendering it completely incompetent with minimal risk of perforation of the vein graft wall. Two methods are available for destruction of valves further down the vein graft: (1) catheter valvulotome; and (2) rigid valvulotome. If the former is chosen, the catheter is passed through the vein from below at this point. The distal end of the saphenous vein is divided, preserving sufficient length to cross the popliteal space to approximate the popliteal artery. A few branches may be divided distally to create the required length and make it more convenient for manipulation of the vein graft during destruction of the valves. The blade is attached and the catheter drawn back so that the valvulotome is completely within the vein graft.

E. The common femoral, superficial femoral, and profunda femoris arteries are occluded with 35-degree peripheral vascular clamps (DeBakey). An arteriotomy is made in the common femoral artery on the anteromedial aspect opposite the origin of the profunda femoris artery. A few of the proximal branches of the saphenous vein may be divided to gain mobility. A lightweight vascular clamp (Diethrich) is used to prevent bleeding from the vein graft.

F. An end-to-side anastomosis of the saphenous vein to the common femoral artery is constructed using continuous stitches of 5/0 polypropylene. The initial five suture loops at the heel of the graft are placed to the distal apex of the arteriotomy before approximating graft to artery. Suturing begins on the side opposite the surgeon. The suture loops are tightened to approximate graft to artery. The suture line is continued in clockwise fashion around the toe of the graft to complete the anastomosis.

G. The vascular clamps are removed from the femoral arteries and blood flow restored to the leg. Blood also flows into the vein graft and distends it until the first competent venous valve is reached. At that point, the valve is set in closed position and the vein graft distal to that point is collapsed. If the catheter valvulotome is used, it is simply pulled through the vein graft by traction on the catheter from below. As competent valves are encountered, the blade cuts cleanly through and the valve is rendered incompetent. The vein graft distends to the next competent valve. Completeness of destruction of valves is demonstrated by vigorous pulsatile blood flow from the vein graft when the catheter valvulotome is competely removed. If the rigid valvulotome is employed, it is passed through a side branch and advanced to a point beyond the most proximal competent valve. The tip is rotated perpendicular to the skin and held against the anterior vein wall. The valvulotome is drawn distally, cutting through the anterior cusps as they are encountered. This procedure is repeated until no further resistance of the valve cusps is encountered. The valvulotome is rotated 180 degrees so that it is oriented posteriorly and the process repeated to destroy the posterior cusps. The valvulotome may be introduced through the end of the vein graft to cut the valves in the distal portion of the vein graft. Pulsatile blood flow from the end of the graft should follow this procedure.

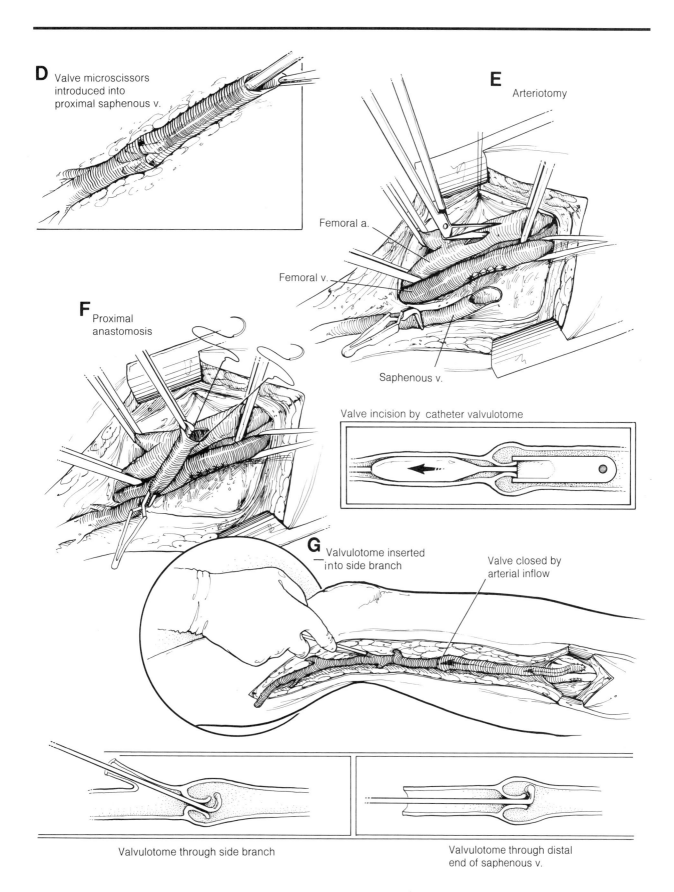

D Valve microscissors introduced into proximal saphenous v.

E Arteriotomy

Femoral a.

Femoral v.

Saphenous v.

F Proximal anastomosis

Valve incision by catheter valvulotome

G Valvulotome inserted into side branch

Valve closed by arterial inflow

Valvulotome through side branch

Valvulotome through distal end of saphenous v.

Femoro-popliteal Artery Bypass

Fig 17–3, H. Retraction devices are placed to expose the contents of the popliteal space.

I. The popliteal artery is isolated between 35-degree angled peripheral vascular clamps (DeBakey). An arteriotomy is made on the antero-medial aspect of the artery. The saphenous vein graft is brought into approximation with the artery and shortened appropriately by cutting a 45-degree bevel.

J. An end-to-side anastomosis of the vein graft to the arteriotomy is constructed using continuous stitches of 6/0 polypropylene. The initial five suture loops are placed at the heel of the graft prior to approximating the graft to the artery at the proximal apex of the arteriotomy. The anastomosis is started at the side opposite the surgeon. The suture loops are tightened to bring the graft to the artery, and the anastomosis is completed in clockwise fashion around the apex of the arteriotomy.

K. Blood flow is established through the bypass graft by removal of the occluding clamp. The foot may be examined to evaluate improvement of arterial flow. Blood flow in the graft and popliteal artery distal to the anastomosis is evaluated with Doppler ultrasound using a sterile probe. The side branches of the saphenous vein graft are ligated with hemoclips. The Doppler probe is used to make sure that continuous flow patterns of arterio-venous fistula are eliminated throughout the length of the graft. The graft is occluded at progressive levels more distally while observing the graft with the Doppler probe. Completion arteriography is performed to evaluate the anastomoses and to be sure that side branches are all ligated.

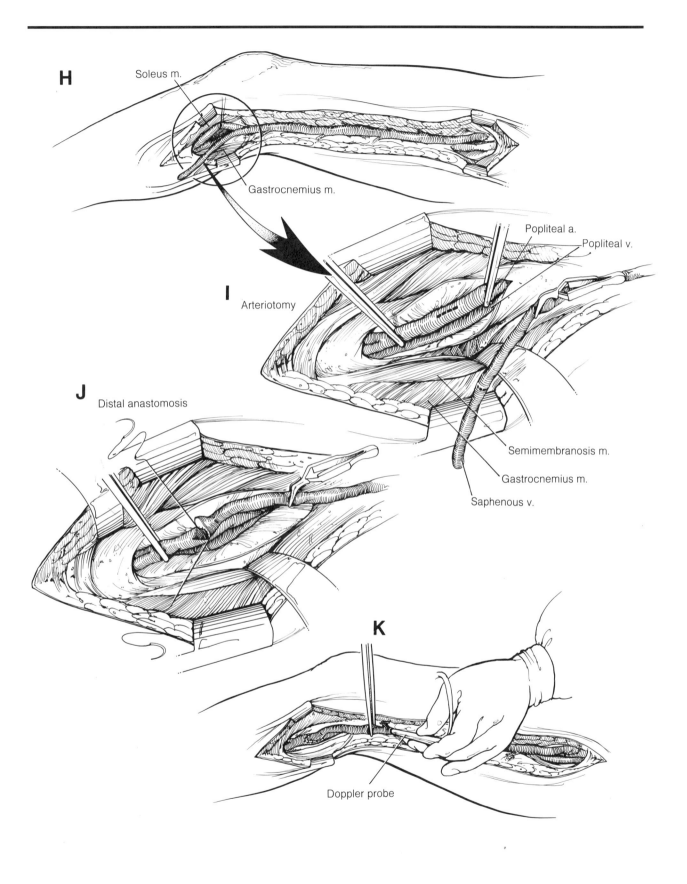

H

Soleus m.

Gastrocnemius m.

I

Arteriotomy

Popliteal a.

Popliteal v.

Semimembranosis m.

Gastrocnemius m.

Saphenous v.

J

Distal anastomosis

K

Doppler probe

18

Femoro-distal Leg Artery Bypass

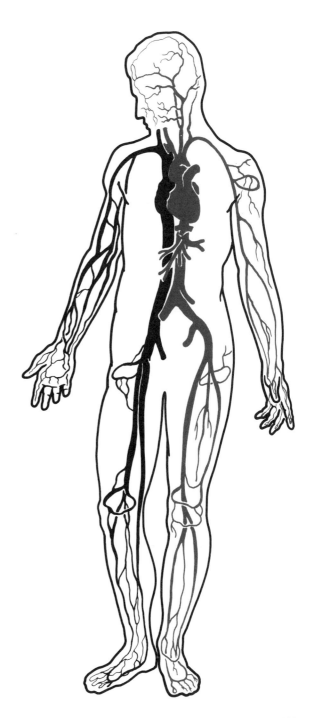

Femoro-posterior Tibial Artery Bypass

Fig 18–1. The anatomic diagrams presented in this chapter to introduce and illustrate the pathology will follow the convention that arteries filled in solid (black) are patent and available for revascularization. This convention is followed for emphasis and clarity of illustration.

Bypass graft from the femoral artery to the posterior tibial artery in the leg below the knee is indicated for limb salvage in patients with ischemic rest pain or gangrene who have suitable anatomy for vascular reconstruction.

A. Arteriography must show evidence of a satisfactory posterior tibial artery that is patent to the pedal arch and unobstructed common femoral artery inflow. There must also be a saphenous vein present that is of good quality. The patient is in the supine position with the abdomen below the umbilicus and the entire leg to the toes in the operating field. The incision is over the course of the saphenous vein extending from the groin to the ankle. The vein is exposed through the course of the incision. This incision will be directly over the posterior tibial artery in the lower calf. The deep fascia is opened above the ankle to expose the artery.

B. Cross-sectional anatomy demonstrates the approach through the deep fascia posterior to the tibia and deep to the flexor digitorum longus muscle and in front of the soleus muscle to the posterior tibial artery.

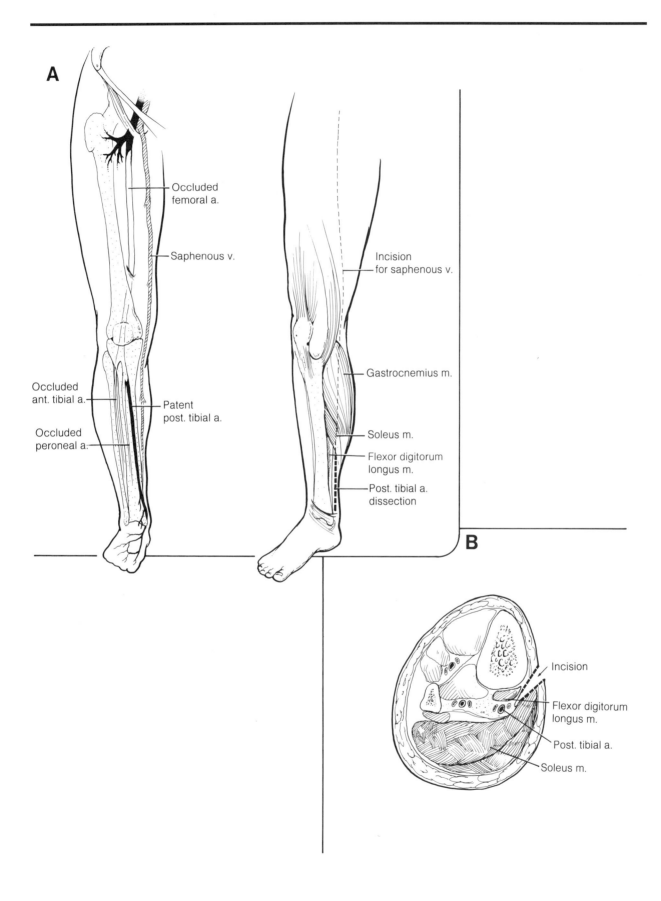

A

Occluded femoral a.

Saphenous v.

Occluded ant. tibial a.

Patent post. tibial a.

Occluded peroneal a.

Incision for saphenous v.

Gastrocnemius m.

Soleus m.

Flexor digitorum longus m.

Post. tibial a. dissection

B

Incision

Flexor digitorum longus m.

Post. tibial a.

Soleus m.

Fig 18–1, C. The deep fascia is opened longitudinally and a self-retaining retractor placed to expose the tissues behind the tibia. Optical loupe magnification (2.5 to 3.5 ×) makes dissection easier. The neurovascular bundle is identified containing the posterior tibial artery, two accompanying veins, and the posterior tibial nerve. Only the anterior surface of the posterior tibial artery is exposed, and it is not elevated from its normal anatomic position in order to maintain stability of the artery and the anastomosis that will be made to it. Care is taken not to tear small crossing vein branches during dissection. Two small areas proximal and distal to the site of proposed anastomosis are freed up alongside the artery to accept the tips of microcoronary bulldog clamps (Dietrich). The accompanying groin dissection is exactly that performed for femoro-popliteal artery bypass graft using in situ saphenous vein. Heparin is administered intravenously to achieve systemic anticoagulant effect. The saphenous vein is anastomosed to the common femoral artery as described for in situ vein bypass graft. The saphenous vein is divided at the ankle, and the valves in the vein are incised using a valvulotome to establish pulsatile arterial flow through the vein graft at the ankle.

D. The microcoronary bulldog clamps are applied to the posterior tibial artery through the small openings alongside the artery. A longitudinal arteriotomy is made using a #15 scalpel blade gently stroked on the surface of the artery until the lumen is entered. The arteriotomy is extended to appropriate length with coronary artery scissors (Potts-Dietrich). The saphenous vein graft is shortened appropriately to approximate the arteriotomy by dividing it, creating a 45-degree bevel at the end. An end-to-side anastomosis of the saphenous vein graft to the posterior tibial artery is constructed by continuous stitches of 6/0 or 7/0 polypropylene suture. The initial five suture loops are placed between the heel of the graft and the proximal apex of the arteriotomy prior to approximating graft to artery. Suturing begins on the side opposite the surgeon. The suture loops are tightened to bring the graft in apposition to the artery. The anastomosis is completed in clockwise fashion around the apex of the arteriotomy. Sutures are placed from the outside aspect of the vein graft and from the intimal surface of the artery.

E. Occluding clamps are removed from the artery and the bypass graft so that blood flow may pass through the anastomosis in the completed repair. Blood flow velocity is evaluated with Doppler ultrasound using a sterile probe in the bypass graft and in the posterior tibial artery distal to the anastomosis. A completion arteriogram is performed. Fascia, subcutaneous tissue, and skin is closed in layers using polyglycolic acid absorbable suture material.

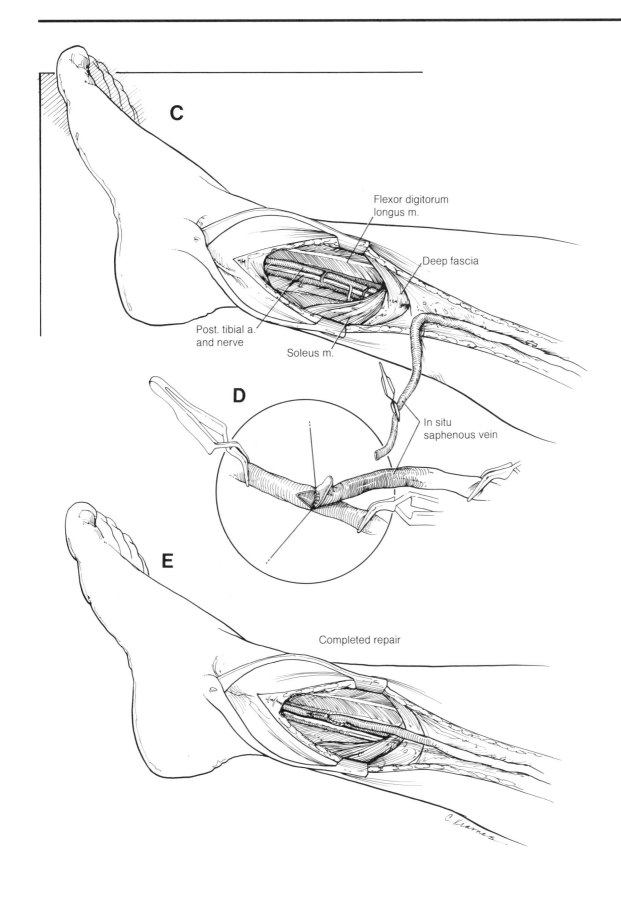

C

Flexor digitorum
longus m.

Deep fascia

Post. tibial a.
and nerve

Soleus m.

D

In situ
saphenous vein

E

Completed repair

C. Krames

Femoro-anterior Tibial Artery Bypass

Fig 18–2. This operation is indicated for limb salvage in patients with ischemic rest pain or gangrene who have suitable anatomy for vascular reconstruction.

A. Arteriography must demonstrate satisfactory anterior tibial artery that is patent to the pedal arch and unobstructed common femoral artery inflow. There must be a good quality saphenous vein. The patient is placed in the supine position on the operating table, and the skin of the abdomen and affected leg to the toes prepared and draped into the operating field. An incision is made in the leg over the course of the greater saphenous vein. This incision is taken over the medial aspect of the leg to a level below the knee corresponding to the expected point of reconstruction to the anterior tibial artery. The saphenous vein is exposed through the entire length of the incision. A second incision is made on the lateral aspect of the leg over the anterior compartment 2 to 3 cm lateral to the tibia and parallel to it.

B. Cross-sectional anatomy demonstrates the incision through the deep fascia into the anterior compartment between the tibialis anterior muscle and the extensor digitorum longus muscle. The anterior tibial artery is located on the interosseous membrane that connects the tibia and fibula.

Femoral, Popliteal, and Tibial Artery Procedures

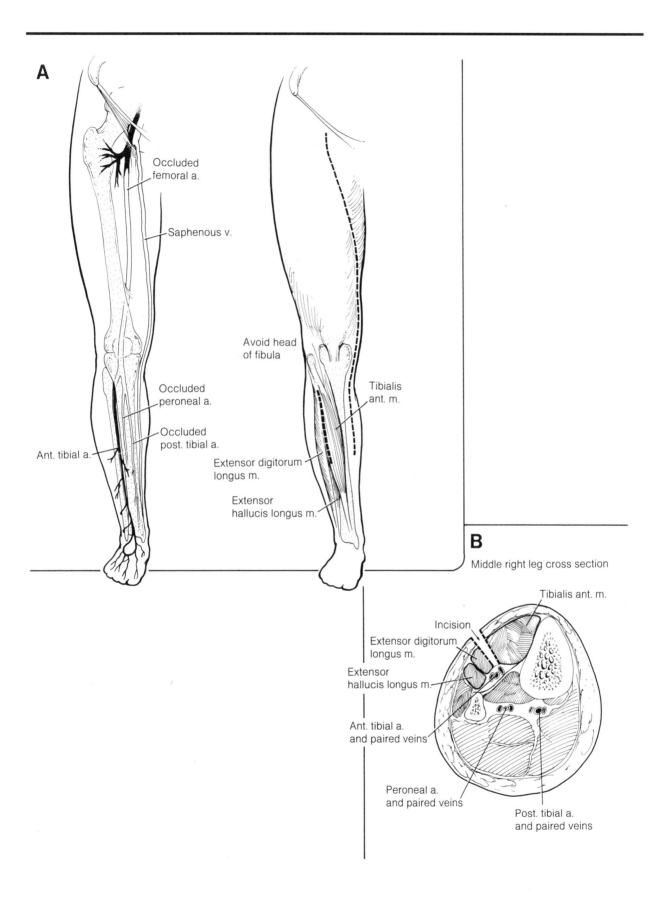

A

Occluded femoral a.

Saphenous v.

Avoid head of fibula

Occluded peroneal a.

Occluded post. tibial a.

Ant. tibial a.

Tibialis ant. m.

Extensor digitorum longus m.

Extensor hallucis longus m.

B

Middle right leg cross section

Tibialis ant. m.

Incision

Extensor digitorum longus m.

Extensor hallucis longus m.

Ant. tibial a. and paired veins

Peroneal a. and paired veins

Post. tibial a. and paired veins

Fig 18–2, C. The knee is flexed over a stack of towels or a rolled sheet. The deep fascia is opened longitudinally and the muscles separated using the handle of a scalpel. Gentle finger dissection is used to further separate the tibialis anterior muscle from the extensor digitorum longus muscle down to the base of the anterior compartment on the interosseous membrane. A self-retaining retractor is placed for exposure. The anterior tibial artery with paired accompanying veins are identified. The peroneal nerve is located lateral to the vascular structures. Only the anterior surface of the artery is cleared by sharp dissection taking care not to elevate it from its vascular bed to maintain stability and to prevent spasm of the artery. Crossing veins must be carefully divided. Two small areas proximal and distal to the proposed site of anastomosis are mobilized alongside the artery for application of the microcoronary bulldog clamps (Diethrich). The dissection of the common femoral artery and vein and anastomosis of the saphenous vein to the femoral artery is exactly that performed for femoro-popliteal artery bypass using in situ saphenous vein. Heparin is administered to the patient prior to any vascular anastomosis. The saphenous vein is divided in the leg preserving sufficient length to cross the interosseous membrane to the lateral aspect of the leg to approximate the anterior tibial artery. A perforation in the interosseous membrane is made for that purpose. A #15 scalpel blade is used to make an incision in the interosseous membrane about 2 cm in length. The valves in the saphenous vein are rendered incompetent and pulsatile blood flow from the end of the graft assured.

D. Microcoronary bulldog clamps are used to occlude a segment of the anterior tibial artery and an arteriotomy made with a #15 scalpel blade. The arteriotomy is extended with coronary artery scissors. The index finger of the left hand is passed through the popliteal space from the medial aspect laterally through the hole in the interosseous membrane. An angled peripheral vascular clamp held in the right hand is guided back from the lateral exposure through the interosseous membrane to the medial surface of the leg. The vein graft is grasped with the clamp. The end of the saphenous vein graft is taken through the opening in the interosseous membrane to the operating field on the lateral aspect of the leg. Care is taken not to twist the graft, and it should be opened to blood flow briefly to assure adequate arterial inflow.

E. The saphenous vein graft is shortened to appropriate length and a 45-degree bevel created at its end. An end-to-side anastomosis of vein graft to anterior tibial artery is constructed using continuous stitches of 6/0 or 7/0 polypropylene. The initial five suture loops are placed at the heel of the graft and the proximal apex of the arteriotomy prior to approximating the graft to the artery. The suture loops are tightened and the remainder of the anastomosis around the distal apex of the arteriotomy completed.

F. The completed repair brings blood flow to the anterior tibial artery via the in situ vein graft across the interosseous membrane. Blood flow is evaluated by Doppler ultrasound and by completion arteriography.

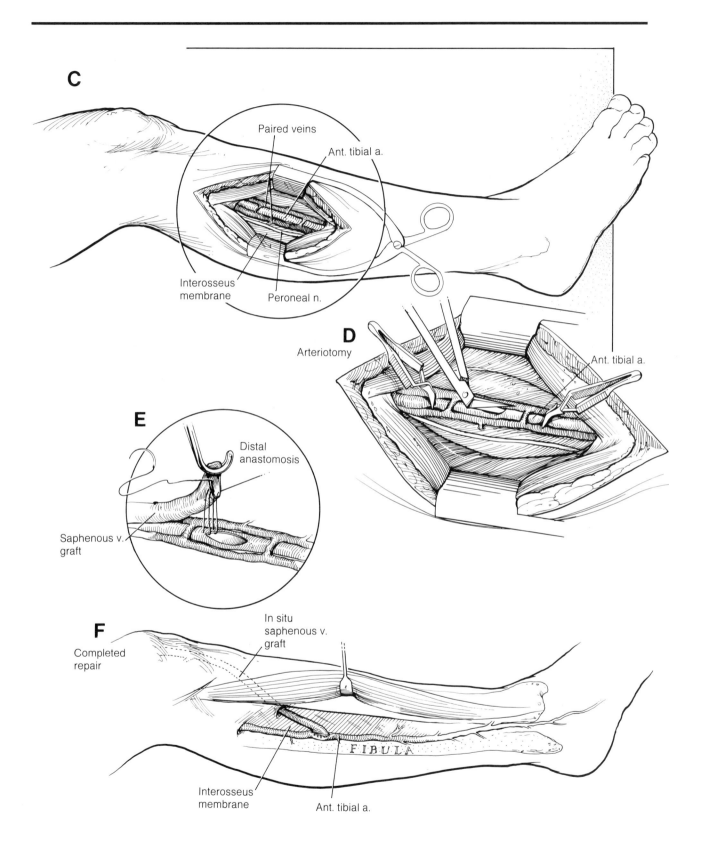

C

Paired veins

Ant. tibial a.

Interosseus membrane

Peroneal n.

D

Arteriotomy

Ant. tibial a.

E

Distal anastomosis

Saphenous v. graft

F

In situ saphenous v. graft

Completed repair

FIBULA

Interosseus membrane

Ant. tibial a.

Femoro-peroneal Artery Bypass

Fig 18–3. This operation is performed for limb salvage in patients with ischemic rest pain or gangrene who have suitable arterial anatomy for vascular reconstruction.

A. Arteriography must demonstrate presence of a satisfactory peroneal artery that communicates with the arterial supply of the foot and unobstructed common femoral arterial inflow. There must be a good saphenous vein present in the leg. The patient is placed in the supine position on the operating table. The skin of the abdomen, leg, and foot to toes is prepared and draped into the operating field. The knee is flexed over a stack of towels or a rolled sheet. An incision is made in the leg over the course of the greater saphenous vein from the groin to the leg below the knee at a level approximating that proposed for distal arterial anastomosis. The saphenous vein is exposed through the length of the incision. The peroneal artery lies deep in the posterior compartment behind the interosseous membrane and closely related to the fibula. It is covered by layers of muscle. The best approach to the artery is from a lateral skin incision directly over the fibula.

B. Cross-sectional anatomy shows how a lateral approach with removal of a segment of the fibula provides access to the peroneal artery through the interosseous membrane which is detached with the bone. Medial approach to this artery is suboptimal because exposure for the anastomosis is compromised.

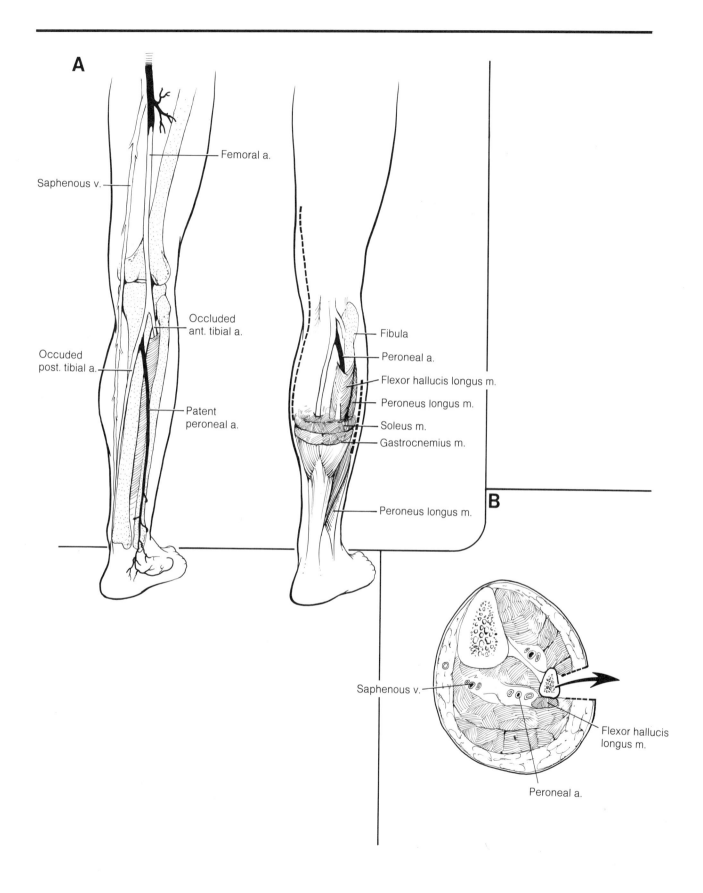

A

Saphenous v.

Femoral a.

Occluded
ant. tibial a.

Occuded
post. tibial a.

Patent
peroneal a.

B

Fibula

Peroneal a.

Flexor hallucis longus m.

Peroneus longus m.

Soleus m.

Gastrocnemius m.

Peroneus longus m.

Saphenous v.

Flexor hallucis
longus m.

Peroneal a.

Fig 18–3, C. The deep fascia over the lateral aspect of the tibia is opened longitudinally. The overlying muscles are separated using the handle of the scalpel. Two self-retaining retractors are used to expose the fibula. About 10 cm of the fibula is cleared of muscle attachment using a periosteal elevator. The fibula is divided at the ends of the exposure using a Gigli or oscillating saw. The interosseous membrane must be released medially to remove this segment of the fibula. The bone fragment is discarded.

D. The peroneal artery with accompanying paired veins is readily exposed once the segment of fibula is removed. The interosseous membrane retracts and the vessels are located in the posterior compartment. Only the anterior aspect of the artery is exposed. A short segment is mobilized alongside the artery proximal and distal to the proposed site of anastomosis to accommodate the tips of the microcoronary bulldog clamps used for occlusion of the artery. Heparin is administered to the patient to achieve systemic anticoagulant effect. Groin dissection and anastomosis of the saphenous vein graft to the common femoral artery is exactly that performed for femoro-popliteal artery bypass using in situ saphenous vein. The saphenous vein is divided distally while preserving sufficient length to reach to the peroneal artery laterally. The valves in the vein graft are rendered incompetent and good arterial inflow assured through the graft. The end of the saphenous vein is guided through the popliteal space to the lateral operating field. This is a simple matter because the interosseous membrane has been detached with resection of the fibula.

E. An arteriotomy is made and the saphenous vein shortened and beveled appropriately. An end-to-side anastomosis of the saphenous vein graft to the peroneal artery is constructed by continuous stitches of 6/0 or 7/0 polypropylene suture. The initial five suture loops are placed at the heel of the graft and the proximal apex of the arteriotomy prior to approximating the tissues. The anastomosis is completed around the distal apex of the arteriotomy.

F. The completed repair brings arterial flow to the peroneal artery via the saphenous vein graft passing from the medial aspect of the leg across the popliteal space to the laterally located artery. Blood flow through the graft and in the peroneal artery distal to the anastomosis is evaluated by Doppler ultrasound and completion arteriography.

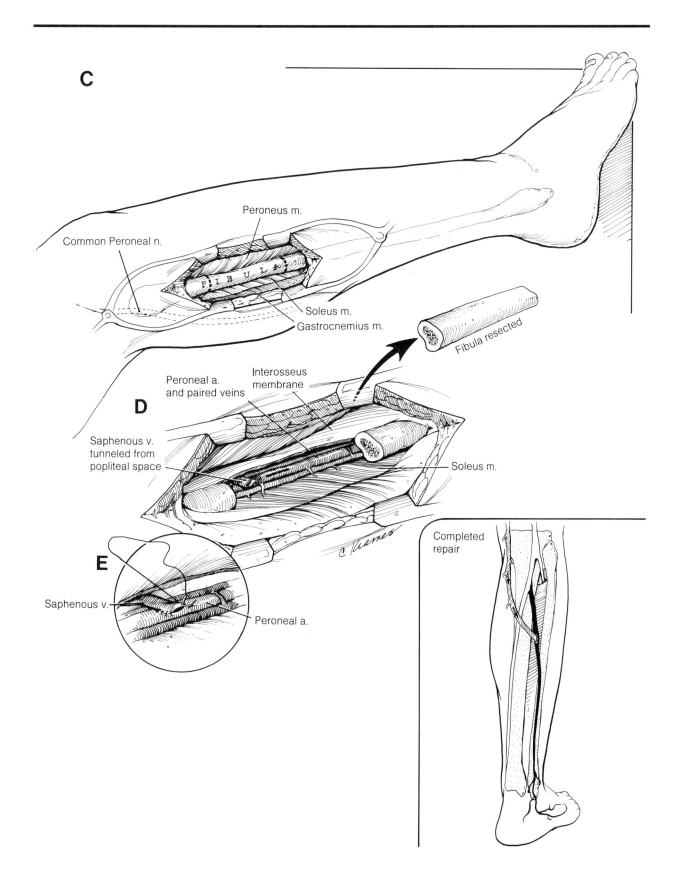

C

Common Peroneal n.

Peroneus m.

FIBULA

Soleus m.

Gastrocnemius m.

Fibula resected

D

Peroneal a.
and paired veins

Interosseus
membrane

Saphenous v.
tunneled from
popliteal space

Soleus m.

c. Thames

E

Completed
repair

Saphenous v.

Peroneal a.

Femoro-dorsalis Pedis Artery Bypass

Fig 18–6. Bypass graft from the femoral artery to the dorsalis pedis artery in the foot is indicated for limb salvage in an occasional patient with ischemic rest pain or gangrene who has suitable anatomy for vascular reconstruction.

A. Arteriography must show evidence of a satisfactory dorsalis pedis artery that communicates with the pedal arch and unobstructed common femoral artery inflow. In most of the patients considered for operation, the common femoral artery will communicate with a normal profunda femoris artery with good thigh collateral. This should be assured because it may be possible to salvage the limb simply with improvement of profunda flow. When profunda flow is good, all branches of the popliteal artery are occluded, and reconstitution of pedal flow is through the dorsalis pedis artery, long distal bypass to foot may be considered.

B. The patient is placed in supine position with the sterile field prepared including the abdomen below the umbilicus, the entire leg, foot, and toes. The incision is directly over saphenous vein from the ankle to the groin. The incision is deviated laterally over the dorsum of the foot to allow for dissection of the dorsalis pedis artery.

C. The saphenous vein may be exposed on the dorsum of the foot and the dorsalis pedis artery mobilized through the primary incision.

D. Cross-sectional anatomy of the foot demonstrates the relationships of the saphenous vein and the dorsalis pedis artery to the first metatarsal bone. The saphenous vein lies in the subcutaneous tissue over the antero-medial aspect of the first metatarsal bone. The dorsalis pedis artery and its accompanying veins are located just below the fascia between the first and second metatarsal bones.

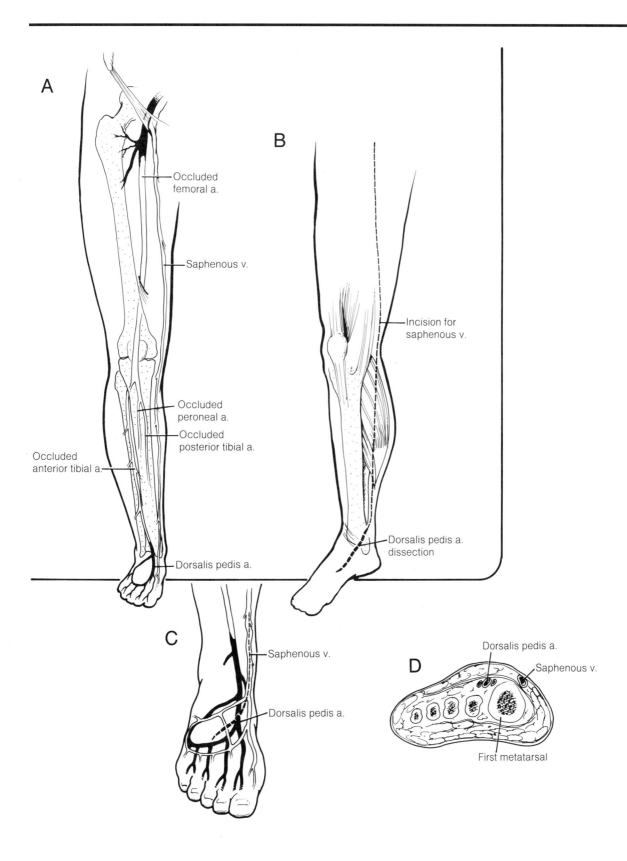

A

Occluded
femoral a.

Saphenous v.

Occluded
peroneal a.

Occluded
posterior tibial a.

Occluded
anterior tibial a.

Dorsalis pedis a.

B

Incision for
saphenous v.

Dorsalis pedis a.
dissection

C

Saphenous v.

Dorsalis pedis a.

D

Dorsalis pedis a.

Saphenous v.

First metatarsal

Fig 18–6, E. The deep fascia is opened longitudinally and a self-retaining retractor placed to expose the tissues between the first and second metatarsal bones. The size of the structures presented in the illustrations are depicted much larger than actual for clarity. The surface of the dorsalis pedis artery is exposed. It is important not to dissect the artery circumferentially or to elevate it from its normal anatomic position so that stability of the artery is maintained and so that the anastomosis of the vein graft to it will also remain stable. The small crossing veins are either not disturbed or carefully ligated or cauterized. Two small areas proximal and distal to the proposed site of anastomosis are freed up alongside the artery to accept the tips of microcoronary bulldog clamps (Dietrich). The accompanying groin dissection is exactly that performed for femoro-popliteal artery bypass graft using in situ saphenous vein graft technique. The saphenous vein is dissected free of the medial aspect of the first metatarsal bone undermining the skin slightly, if necessary. The vein is divided preserving sufficient length to cross over to the dorsalis pedis artery after heparin is administered to achieve systemic anticoagulant effect. A catheter valvulotome is passed through the saphenous vein to the groin. The saphenous vein is anastomosed to the common femoral artery as described for in situ vein bypass graft. The valvulotome is pulled back through the vein to incise all of the valves and establish pulsatile arterial flow through the vein graft to the foot.

F. Microcoronary bulldog clamps are applied to the dorsalis pedis artery through the small openings alongside the artery. A longitudinal arteriotomy is made using a #15 scalpel blade gently stroked on the surface of the artery until the lumen is entered. The arteriotomy is extended to appropriate length with coronary artery scissors (Potts-Dietrich). The saphenous vein graft is shortened appropriately to approximate the dorsalis pedis artery, creating a 45-degree bevel at the end as it is divided.

G. An end-to-side anastomosis of the saphenous vein graft to the posterior tibial artery is constructed by continuous stitches of 7/0 polypropylene suture. The initial five suture loops are placed between the heel of the graft and the proximal apex of the arteriotomy. The suture loops are pulled up to bring the graft in apposition with the artery. This separates the edges of the arteriotomy and provides good exposure of the distal apex of the arteriotomy for suture placement.

H. The completed anastomosis brings blood flow through the saphenous vein bypass graft to the pedal arch. Blood flow velocity is evaluated with Doppler ultrasound using a sterile probe. A completion arteriogram is performed. The subcutaneous tissue and skin are closed in layers with polyglycolic acid absorbable suture material. Pulsation in the bypass graft is easily palpable through the skin on the dorsum of the foot just below the ankle.

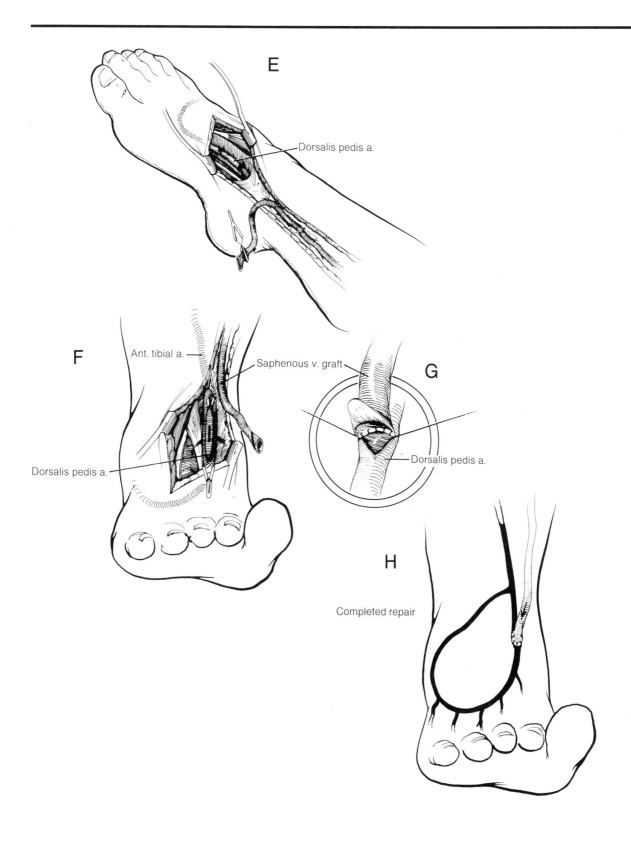

E — Dorsalis pedis a.

F — Ant. tibial a. — Saphenous v. graft — Dorsalis pedis a.

G — Dorsalis pedis a.

H — Completed repair

Sequential Femoro-popliteal-posterior Tibial Artery Bypass

Fig 18–4. This operation is performed for limb salvage in patients with ischemic rest pain or gangrene with arterial anatomy suitable for vascular reconstruction. The theory of using sequential anastomoses is that greater run-off through the bypass graft may enhance total limb blood flow and prolong the patency of the graft.

A. Arteriography must show evidence for patent posterior tibial artery in communication with the pedal arch, an isolated patent segment of the popliteal artery, and unobstructed common femoral artery inflow. A suitable saphenous vein graft must be available. The patient is in the supine position with the skin of the abdomen and the entire leg prepared and draped into the operating field. The knee is flexed over a stack of towels or a rolled sheet. A reversed saphenous vein graft is employed. The incision is directly over the saphenous vein extending from groin to ankle. Deep fascial incisions are made via the primary skin incision at the knee to expose the popliteal artery and above the ankle to expose the posterior tibial artery. The femoral arteries are exposed at the groin. The saphenous vein is removed from the length of the incision and prepared for bypass graft in the usual fashion by attachment of an irrigation needle or cannula and gentle distension to check for completeness of ligation of branches.

B. The posterior tibial artery is exposed, and only its anterior surface is dissected for anastomosis. Heparin is administered intravenously to achieve systemic anticoagulant effect. A short segment of the artery is isolated between microcoronary bulldog clamps (Diethrich). A longitudinal arteriotomy is made. An end-to-side anastomosis of the reversed saphenous vein to the posterior tibial artery is constructed using continuous stitches of 6/0 or 7/0 polypropylene. The initial five suture loops are placed at the heel of the graft and the proximal apex of the arteriotomy. The remainder of the anastomosis is completed after pulling up the suture loops by continuous stitch around the distal apex of the arteriotomy. Removal of occlusion clamps allow the collateral blood flow to fill the posterior tibial artery and the vein graft to the first competent valve.

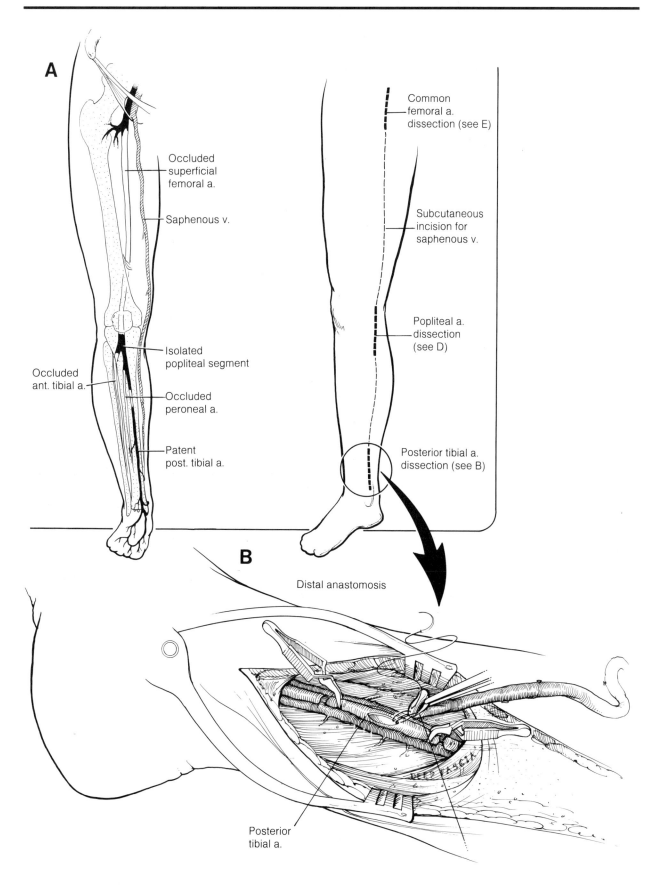

A

Occluded
superficial
femoral a.

Saphenous v.

Occluded
ant. tibial a.

Isolated
popliteal segment

Occluded
peroneal a.

Patent
post. tibial a.

Common
femoral a.
dissection (see E)

Subcutaneous
incision for
saphenous v.

Popliteal a.
dissection
(see D)

Posterior tibial a.
dissection (see B)

B

Distal anastomosis

Posterior
tibial a.

Fig 18–4, C. A tunneling device is used to create a passageway below the deep fascia to the popliteal space between the heads of the gastrocnemius muscle. The saphenous vein graft is attached to the tunneler by the irrigating device and distended gently by irrigating solution. The tunneler is withdrawn proximally pulling the saphenous vein through the passageway to approximate the popliteal artery. Care must be taken to avoid twisting the graft.

D. The popliteal artery is exposed and a short segment isolated between 35-degree angled peripheral vascular clamps (DeBakey) or a single curved vascular clamp (Derra). This segment of artery should be the most nearly normal that can be identified in the popliteal space. A longitudinal arteriotomy is made in the popliteal artery. As the vein graft is distended with irrigating solution, a corresponding longitudinal venotomy is made in the saphenous vein graft as it approximates the location of the incision made in the popliteal artery. A side-to-side anastomosis of the saphenous vein graft to the popliteal artery is constructed by continuous stitches of 5/0 or 6/0 polypropylene suture. Stitches are passed from the outside of the vein graft and from the intimal surface (inside) of the artery. The initial five suture loops at the distal end of the arteriotomy are placed prior to approximating the tissues. The suture loops are tightened and the anastomosis completed around the proximal apex of the arteriotomy.

E. The tunneling device is passed from the groin to the popliteal fossa beneath the sartorius muscle. The vein graft is attached to the tunneling device by the irrigating cannula and gently distended to remove twisting of the graft. The vein graft is pulled through the passageway in the thigh to the groin by removal of the tunneler with care taken not to twist the graft. A final check of graft function is made by gentle distension and irrigation of the graft. The common femoral artery is isolated by vascular clamps. An arteriotomy is made opposite the origin of the profunda femoris artery. The saphenous vein graft is shortened, beveled, and cut back appropriately to approximate and cover the arteriotomy in the femoral artery. An end-to-side anastomosis of the saphenous vein graft to the femoral artery is constructed using 5/0 polypropylene. The initial five suture loops are placed between the heel of the graft and the distal apex of the arteriotomy beginning at the side opposite the surgeon prior to approximating the tissues. The suture loops are tightened and the anastomosis completed by continuous suture technique around the proximal apex of the arteriotomy.

F. Vascular occlusion clamps are removed and blood flow established through the completed bypass graft to the leg. Blood flow velocity is evaluated using Doppler ultrasound and completion arteriography.

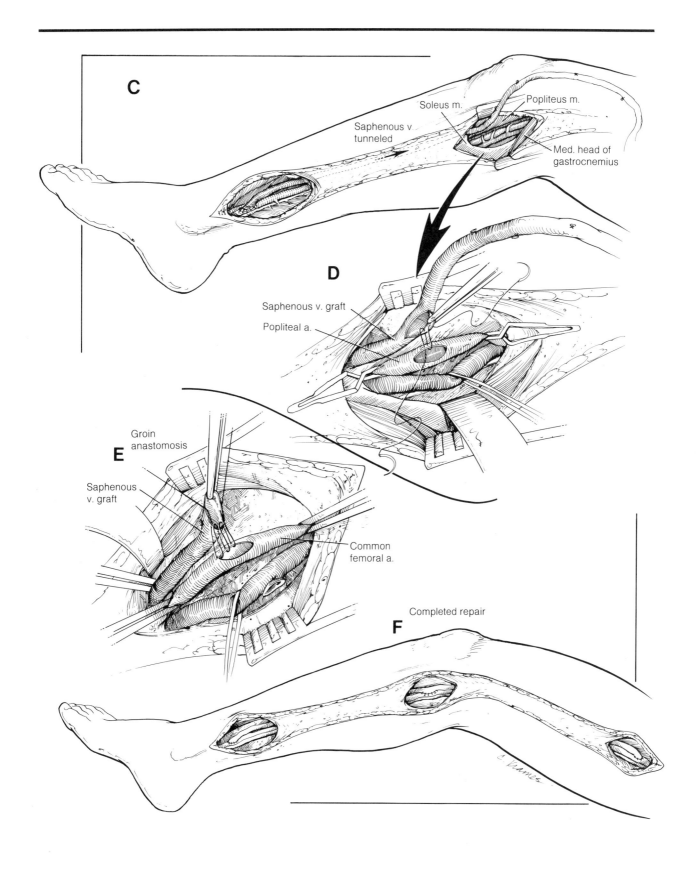

C

Saphenous v tunneled

Soleus m.

Popliteus m.

Med. head of gastrocnemius

D

Saphenous v. graft

Popliteal a.

E

Groin anastomosis

Saphenous v. graft

Common femoral a.

F

Completed repair

Composite Graft Procedures for Insufficient Saphenous Vein

Femoro-popliteal-posterior Tibial Artery: Composite Sequential Bypass Graft

Fig 18–5. Composite graft procedures are indicated for limb salvage in patients with ischemic rest pain or gangrene when there is not sufficient suitable saphenous vein for bypass graft. Arteriography must demonstrate that the posterior tibial artery is patent to the pedal arch, an isolated patent popliteal artery segment is present, and there is unobstructed common femoral artery inflow.

A. The patient is placed in the supine position with the skin of the abdomen, leg, and foot prepared and draped into the operating field. The skin incision is started in the groin over the origin of the saphenous vein. The incision is continued down the leg over the course of the greater saphenous vein. Should the vein become unsuitable for bypass graft at some point in the thigh, the decision to proceed with composite graft is made. The femoral artery is exposed through the primary skin incision in the groin. The available saphenous vein is removed from the thigh. The popliteal artery is exposed through a separate incision on the medial aspect of the leg. The posterior tibial artery is exposed through a separate incision above the ankle. Heparin is administered intravenously to achieve systemic anticoagulant effect. A segment of the popliteal artery is isolated between vascular clamps and a longitudinal incision made into it. A polytetrafluoroethylene (PTFE) graft 6 to 8 mm in diameter is chosen for bypass from femoral artery to the popliteal artery. The graft is placed flat on a towel and cut obliquely with a fresh #11 scalpel blade. An end-to-side anastomosis of the graft to the popliteal artery is constructed by continuous stitch using 5/0 or 6/0 polypropylene or PTFE suture. The anastomosis is constructed in the standard fashion placing the initial five suture loops at the heel of the graft, tightening the loops, and completing the suture line around the distal apex of the arteriotomy.

B. A tunnel is created between the popliteal fossa and the groin deep to the sartorius muscle. The prosthetic graft is pulled through the passageway to the groin. The common femoral artery is isolated by vascular clamps and an arteriotomy made opposite the origin of the profunda femoris artery. An end-to-side anastomosis of the prosthetic bypass graft to the common femoral artery is constructed using 5/0 polypropylene or PTFE suture. The heel of the graft is attached by loose suture loops initially. The suture loops are tightened to approximate graft to artery and the remainder of the anastomosis completed around the proximal apex of the arteriotomy.

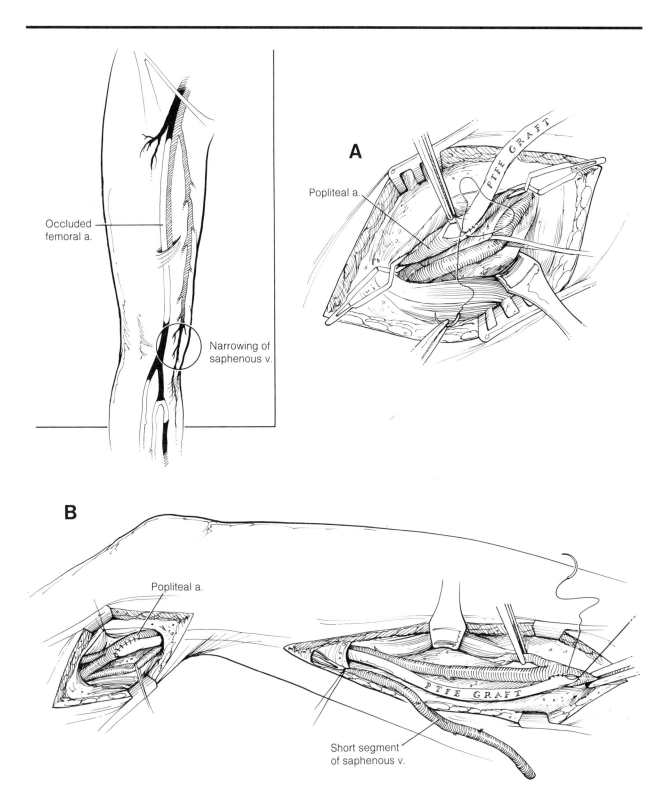

A

Popliteal a.

PTFE GRAFT

B

Popliteal a.

PTFE GRAFT

Short segment
of saphenous v.

Occluded
femoral a.

Narrowing of
saphenous v.

Fig 18–5, C. An anastomosis of the reversed saphenous vein graft is made to an arteriotomy in the posterior tibial artery above the ankle in standard fashion as previously described. A tunnel is created beneath the deep fascia from the ankle to the popliteal space between the heads of the gastrocnemius muscle. The saphenous vein graft is attached to the tunneler device and distended gently to prevent twisting as it is pulled through the passageway in the leg to the popliteal space.

D. An opening is made into the prosthetic graft just above the anastomosis to the popliteal artery. An end-to-side anastomosis of the saphenous vein graft to the prosthetic graft is constructed using 6/0 polypropylene or PTFE suture.

The completed repair brings blood flow to the leg via prosthetic bypass graft to the isolated popliteal segment and by saphenous vein bypass graft to the distal posterior tibial artery. While not as satisfactory in terms of late patency as a bypass graft constructed entirely of saphenous vein, this type of reconstruction should be better than bypass graft using prosthetic material alone.

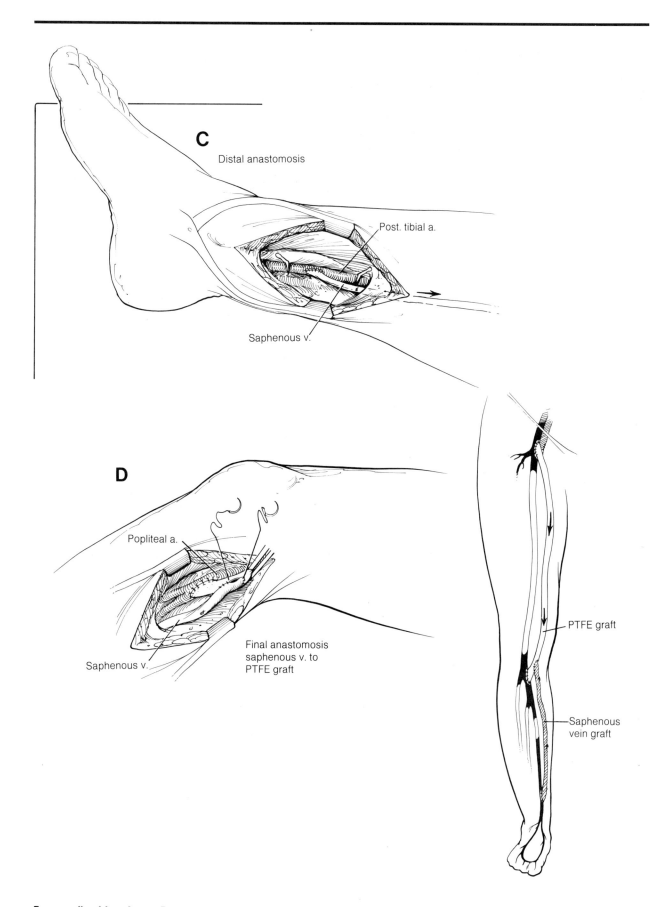

C

Distal anastomosis

Post. tibial a.

Saphenous v.

D

Popliteal a.

Saphenous v.

Final anastomosis
saphenous v. to
PTFE graft

PTFE graft

Saphenous
vein graft

Composite Femoral Artery and Saphenous Vein Bypass Graft

Fig 18–7. When the saphenous vein is found to be unsatisfactory for bypass from the femoral artery to the popliteal artery because it becomes too small at some level in the thigh, the available segment of vein may be sufficient, provided some extension can be made to lengthen the common femoral artery. Composite prosthetic grafts have been used but are not completely satisfactory. Endarterectomy of a portion of the superficial femoral artery may provide sufficient length to attach to the saphenous vein segment to allow it to reach the desired point in the popliteal artery.

A. An incision is made in the leg beginning over the origin of the saphenous vein and extended over the course of the vein to a point where it becomes unsatisfactory for use as a bypass graft. The available segment of saphenous vein is removed from the leg and prepared for bypass grafting in the usual manner. The common femoral, superficial femoral, and profunda femoris arteries are exposed and controlled. The superficial femoral artery is exposed as it courses beneath the sartorius muscle toward the adductor canal. Heparin is administered intravenously to achieve systemic anticoagulant effect. The common femoral and profunda femoris arteries are occluded by angled peripheral vascular clamps. The superficial femoral artery is ligated and divided as it enters the adductor canal at a point that provides sufficient length when combined with the saphenous vein to reach the popliteal artery.

B. An arteriotomy is made in the common femoral artery opposite the origin of the profunda femoris artery. A Freer septum elevator is used to separate the atherosclerotic intima-media from the adventitia of the common femoral artery and the superficial femoral artery.

C. The atherosclerotic core is separated from the arteries and a clean, tapered endpoint assured in the profunda femoris artery.

D. The arteriotomy in the common femoral artery is closed by direct suture using 5/0 or 6/0 polypropylene. An end-to-end anastomosis of the reversed saphenous vein graft to the endarterectomized superficial femoral artery is constructed using continuous stitches of 6/0 polypropylene suture.

The saphenous vein graft is continued to the popliteal space where an end-to-side anastomosis is constructed to the popliteal artery. The composite graft provides blood flow to the leg through the saphenous vein graft across the knee joint by extension from the superficial femoral artery.

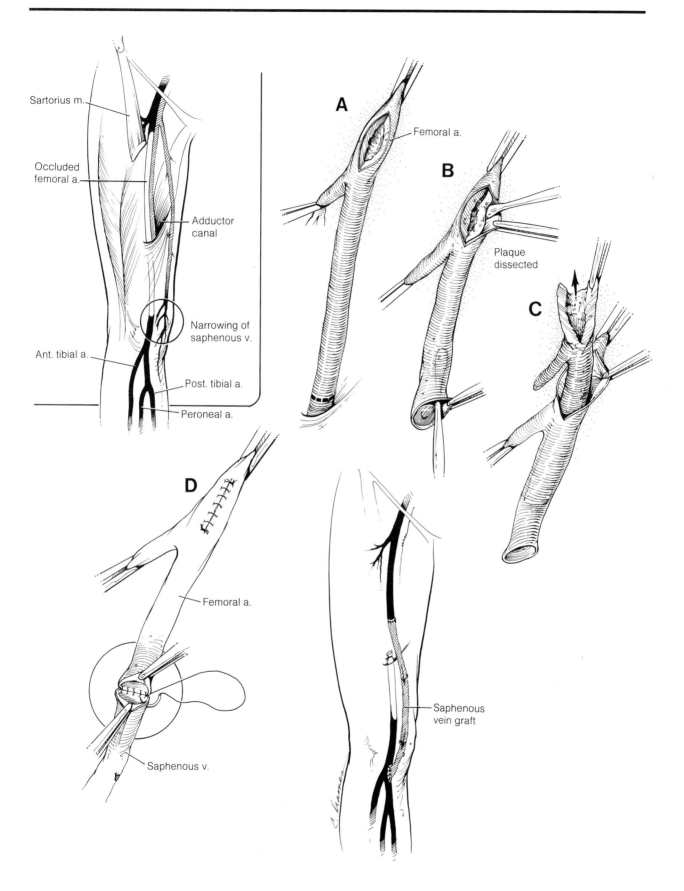

Sartorius m.

Occluded femoral a.

Adductor canal

Narrowing of saphenous v.

Ant. tibial a.

Post. tibial a.

Peroneal a.

A

Femoral a.

B

Plaque dissected

C

D

Femoral a.

Saphenous v.

Saphenous vein graft

Popliteal Aneurysm

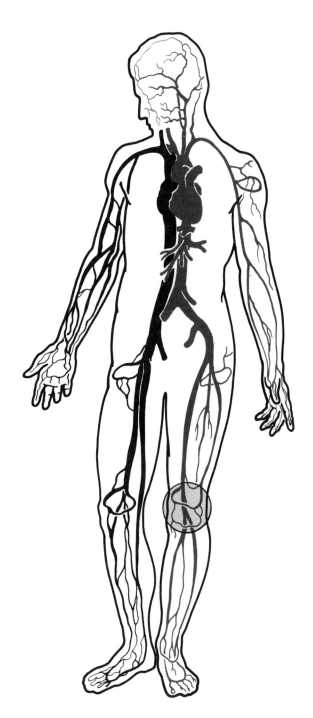

19

Fig 19–1. Aneurysm of the popliteal artery frequently presents with thrombotic occlusion of the popliteal embolism to the distal arteries of the foot. The essential principle of repair of popliteal aneurysm is the exclusion of the aneurysm from the distal blood flow pathway to remove the possibility of embolism of debris of the aneurysm contents. How this is accomplished depends on the actual pathology encountered.

A. For small aneurysm of the popliteal artery, the artery is divided at the termination of the aneurysmal portion and distal circulation restored via an in situ saphenous vein graft. The popliteal artery is ligated above the aneurysm to totally exclude it and allow it to heal by thrombosis and organization of clot.

B. Large aneurysm of the popliteal artery is treated by more conventional aneurysm resection technique. The popliteal artery is opened and an end-to-end interposition of a reversed saphenous vein graft is used to replace the aneurysmal segment of the artery.

C. When popliteal aneurysm accompanies ectasia of the superficial femoral artery, the popliteal artery is divided and distal circulation restored via an in situ saphenous vein graft. The aneurysmal portion may be removed and the end of the superficial femoral artery closed to prevent further embolus from the ectatic portion of the artery.

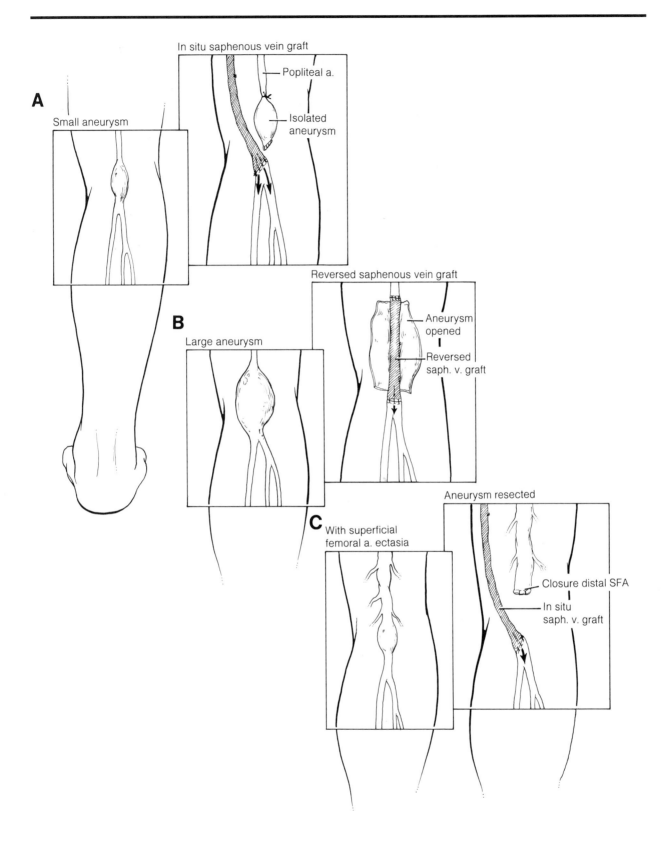

A

Small aneurysm

In situ saphenous vein graft

Popliteal a.

Isolated aneurysm

B

Large aneurysm

Reversed saphenous vein graft

Aneurysm opened

Reversed saph. v. graft

C

With superficial femoral a. ectasia

Aneurysm resected

Closure distal SFA

In situ saph. v. graft

Fig 19–1, D. An incision is made on the medial aspect of the leg. The incision should be at the posterior edge of the condyle of the femur and should span the knee joint.

E. The incision comes down over the tendinous attachments of the sartorius, gracilis, semimembranous, and semitendinosus muscles and the gastrocnemius muscle just below. The greater saphenous vein is located in the subcutaneous tissues, usually on the posterior edge of the incision. If the vein is of adequate diameter at this level, it may be used for the reconstruction. Otherwise, a separate incision in the groin is required to obtain vein of larger caliber.

F. The tendinous attachments of the muscles are released to gain access to the popliteal fossa. The popliteal aneurysm is identified and partially freed up to be able to identify the normal portions of artery entering and leaving the aneurysm. Distal control of the popliteal artery should be accomplished as soon as possible. The aneurysm should be manipulated minimally to prevent dislodgment of debris with consequent embolus to the foot circulation.

Popliteal aneurysm - surgical approach:

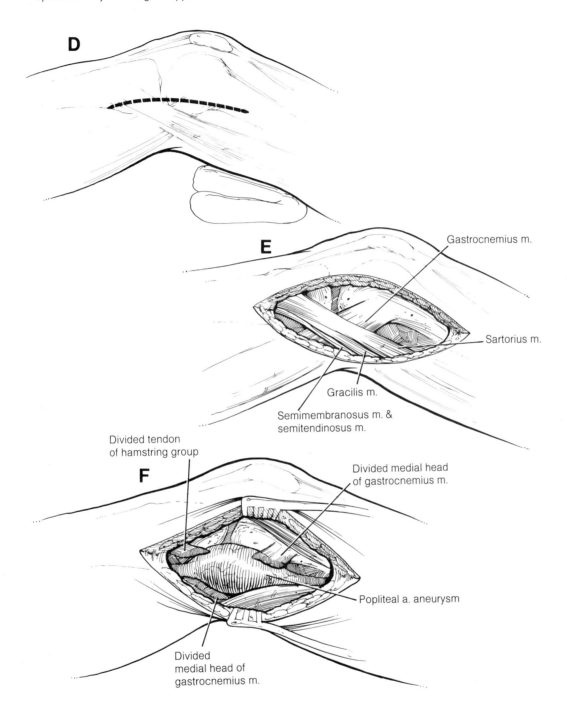

D

E

Gastrocnemius m.

Sartorius m.

Gracilis m.

Semimembranosus m. &
semitendinosus m.

Divided tendon
of hamstring group

F

Divided medial head
of gastrocnemius m.

Popliteal a. aneurysm

Divided
medial head of
gastrocnemius m.

Fig 19–1, G. Vascular occlusion clamps are applied to the normal popliteal artery distal and proximal to the aneurysm. A longitudinal incision is made into the aneurysm. Contained clot and debris are removed by endarterectomy.

H. Bleeding from any patent branches of the popliteal artery in the aneurysmal portion is controlled by simply oversewing the orifices of the branches. The popliteal artery is divided proximal and distal to the aneurysm, leaving the opened aneurysm in situ. The aneurysm is not excised in order to prevent injury to the nerves and veins of the popliteal fossa that are often attached by inflammatory fibrous tissue to the aneurysm.

I. A segment of saphenous vein is excised, all side branches ligated, and prepared for replacement graft. The vein graft is reversed and the ends cut back (spatulated) to account for disparity in diameter compared to the end of the popliteal artery. An end-to-end anastomosis of the vein graft to the popliteal artery is constructed using continuous stitches of 6/0 polypropylene suture.

J. The completed vein graft interposition restores blood flow to the distal popliteal artery. The aneurysm wall is simply allowed to lie around the graft without closure as the incision is repaired.

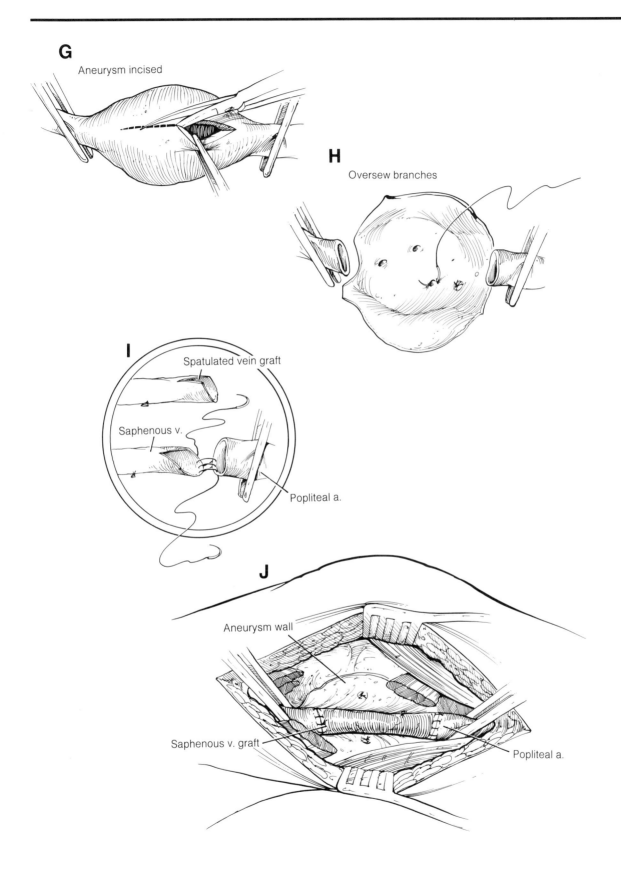

G

Aneurysm incised

H

Oversew branches

I

Spatulated vein graft

Saphenous v.

Popliteal a.

J

Aneurysm wall

Saphenous v. graft

Popliteal a.

Popliteal Artery Entrapment

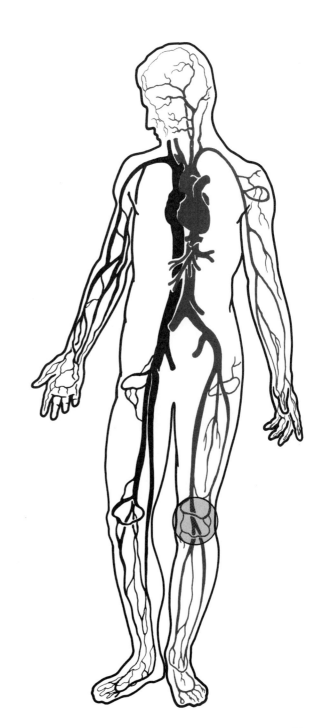

20

Fig 20–1. Popliteal artery entrapment typically presents in young men as unilateral calf claudication. Bilateral symptomatic popliteal artery entrapment may occur less commonly. The basic anomaly is compression of the popliteal artery by the medial head of the gastrocnemius muscle. This causes chronic intermittent arterial trauma, resulting in gradual thickening and fibrotic changes in the arterial wall that progress to stenosis or thrombosis of the popliteal artery. A physical finding suggestive of the diagnosis is disappearance of pedal pulses with dorsiflexion of the foot.

A. *Normal anatomy, posterior view, right leg.* The normal course of the popliteal artery is between the medial and lateral heads of the gastrocnemius muscle as they attach to the femoral condyles. The popliteal vein and tibial nerve are closely related to the popliteal artery as it courses through the popliteal space.

B. *Type I anatomy.* The most common anatomic arrangement of the anomaly is compression of a medially displaced popliteal artery by the medial head of the gastrocnemius muscle. This arrangement accounts for three fourths of all cases. Type I anatomy consists of medial deviation of the course of the popliteal artery so that it passes medially around the medial head of the gastrocnemius that is normally inserted onto the medial condyle of the femur.

C. *Type II anatomy.* This anomaly consists of popliteal artery compression due to its medial displacement by the medial head of the gastrocnemius muscle which is inserted on the medial condyle of the femur more lateral than normal.

D. *Type III anatomy.* This anomaly consists of compression of the popliteal artery in its usual course across the popliteal fossa by an accessory slip of the gastrocnemius muscle or tendinous insertion laterally to the medial condyle of the femur. It is distinguished by the normal course of the popliteal artery on angiograms from the Type I and II anomalies that show medial deviation of the popliteal artery.

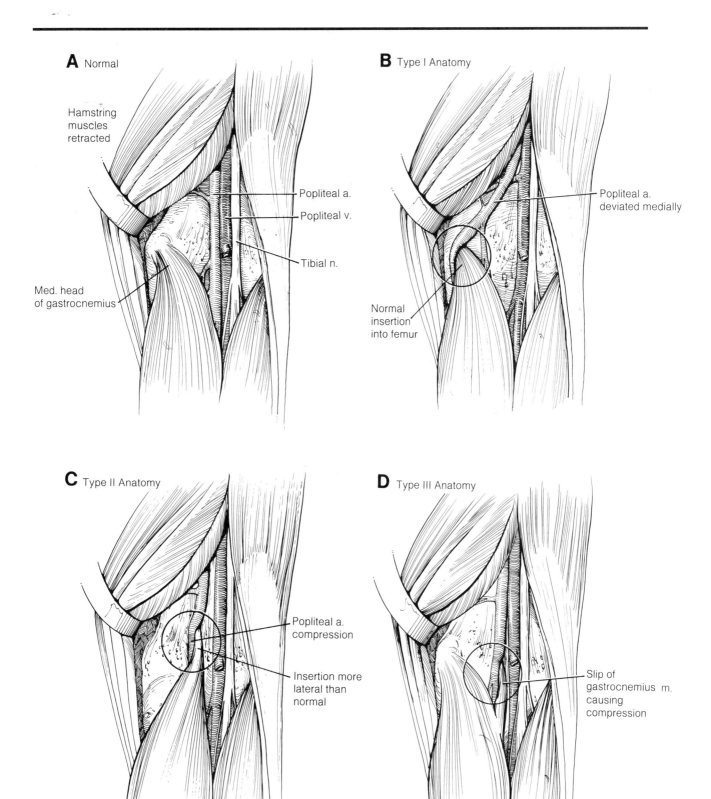

A Normal

Hamstring muscles retracted

Med. head of gastrocnemius

Popliteal a.

Popliteal v.

Tibial n.

B Type I Anatomy

Popliteal a. deviated medially

Normal insertion into femur

C Type II Anatomy

Popliteal a. compression

Insertion more lateral than normal

D Type III Anatomy

Slip of gastrocnemius m. causing compression

Popliteal Artery Entrapment

Fig 20–2. Operative approach for popliteal artery entrapment is through a posterior popliteal fossa incision with the patient in the prone position on the operating table. This greatly improves the exposure and evaluation of the course of the popliteal artery and its relationship to the medial head of the gastrocnemius muscle compared to the usual medial approach to the popliteal artery. An "S"-shaped incision is made beginning superior and medial to the popliteal fossa, extending the incision transversely across the popliteal fossa, and curving inferior to the lateral aspect of the leg below the fossa. This reduces probability of flexion contracture with wound healing.

A. The deep fascia is incised longitudinally. The popliteal artery, vein, and accompanying tibial nerve are identified at the exit from the adductor canal. The popliteal artery is exposed to the point that it passes beneath the medial head of the gastrocnemius muscle. The muscle overlying the artery is carefully separated from the popliteal artery. A right angle clamp is used to elevate the muscle away from the vessel. The muscle is divided by cautery blade.

B. The popliteal artery is carefully examined after it has been freed from muscle entrapment and allowed to return to normal position. Operative arteriography is performed. If the popliteal artery is found to be normal, nothing further needs to be done.

C. In most cases, the popliteal artery will be stenosed or thrombosed so that reconstructive operation is required. The involved segment should be resected and replaced with an interposition of saphenous vein graft attached in end-to-end fashion to the popliteal artery proximally and distally. The anastomoses are constructed with continuous suture technique using 6/0 polypropylene. The medial head of the gastrocnemius muscle may be reapproximated.

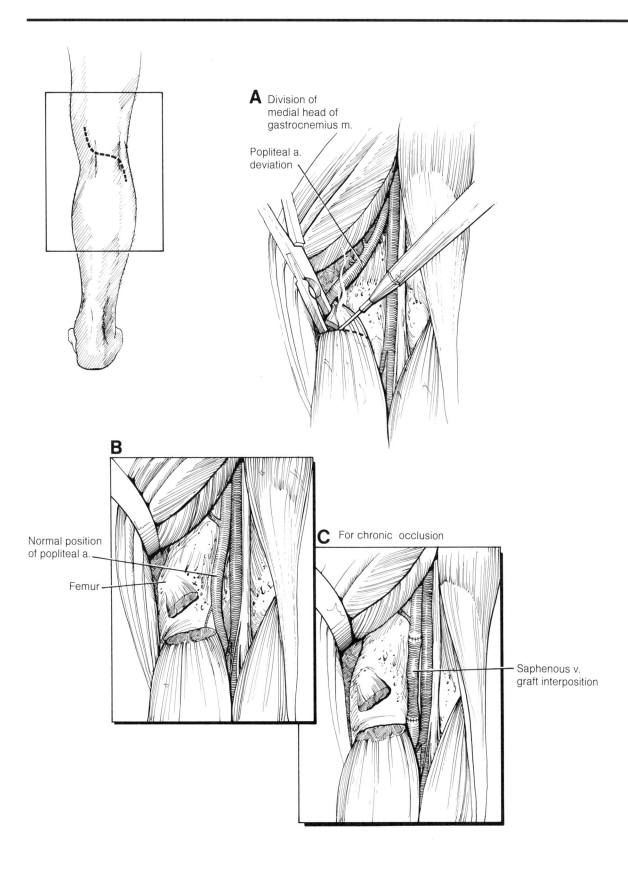

A Division of medial head of gastrocnemius m.

Popliteal a. deviation

B

Normal position of popliteal a.

Femur

C For chronic occlusion

Saphenous v. graft interposition

Abdominal Aortic Aneurysm (Infrarenal)

21

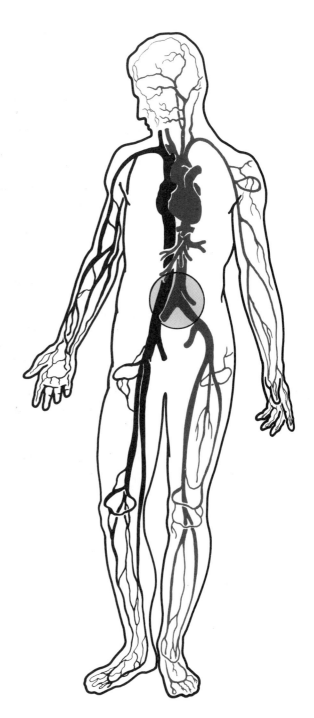

Fig 21-1. A midline incision is made that extends from the xyphoid process of the sternum to the pubic ramus. The urinary bladder should have been emptied by Foley catheter drainage and the bowel contents removed by laxative and enema. A self-retaining ring retractor that attaches to the operating table (Wilkinson) is very helpful and reduces the number of assistants required to obtain good exposure of the abdominal aorta in the retroperitoneal space. The transverse colon and attached omentum are retracted from the abdomen and placed on moist laparotomy sponges on the anterior chest wall. The small bowel is eviscerated and retracted to expose the base of the mesentery.

A. An incision is made in the posterior peritoneum over the aneurysmal abdominal aorta. The incision is extended proximally alongside the fourth portion of the duodenum while preserving the inferior mesenteric vein and the middle colic artery. The incision is taken inferiorly over the right common iliac artery. Only minimal dissection of the anterior surface of the aneurysm is required. The base of the small bowel mesentery is mobilized to the right of the anterior surface of the aorta. The small bowel is contained in a plastic bag (Lahey) and retracted to the right, outside the abdominal cavity. The splenic flexure of the colon is packed away and retracted. Three moist towels are placed to cover the small bowel and colon in preparation for placement of retractors. The self-retaining retractor will maintain the exposure with only occasional manual retraction required to expose the proximal neck of the aneurysm.

B. Proximal control of the aorta is the initial step of the dissection of the aneurysm. The left renal vein is identified and minimally exposed. The aorta is controlled just below the vein. Generally, there is sufficient uninvolved aorta below the renal arteries to allow control without compromising blood flow to the kidneys. The aneurysmal portion of the aorta will usually lift the neck of the aneurysm away from the spine so that there is a space between the uninvolved aorta and the anterior surface of the spinal column where safe control is readily achieved. With minimal interruption of tissues alongside the aorta, it is possible to place a curved clamp (Shall-Cross) behind the aorta. Gentle manipulation with the index finger is a useful aid to the dissection. Distal control of the aorta is accomplished on the proximal common iliac arteries. Minimal dissection of the arteries at their sides is all that is required. It is not advisable to attempt to completely encircle the arteries to avoid injury to the iliac veins that are often intimately attached to the posterior aspect of the arteries.

Heparin, 100–200 units/kg, is administered intravenously to the patient. Alternatively, the procedure may be performed in selected cases with regional heparinization of the legs by injection of heparinized saline into the iliac arteries just as the aorta is isolated and blood flow interrupted to the legs. This method requires expeditious surgery in order to decrease the risk of thrombosis in the lower extremities.

Aneurysm of Abdominal Aorta

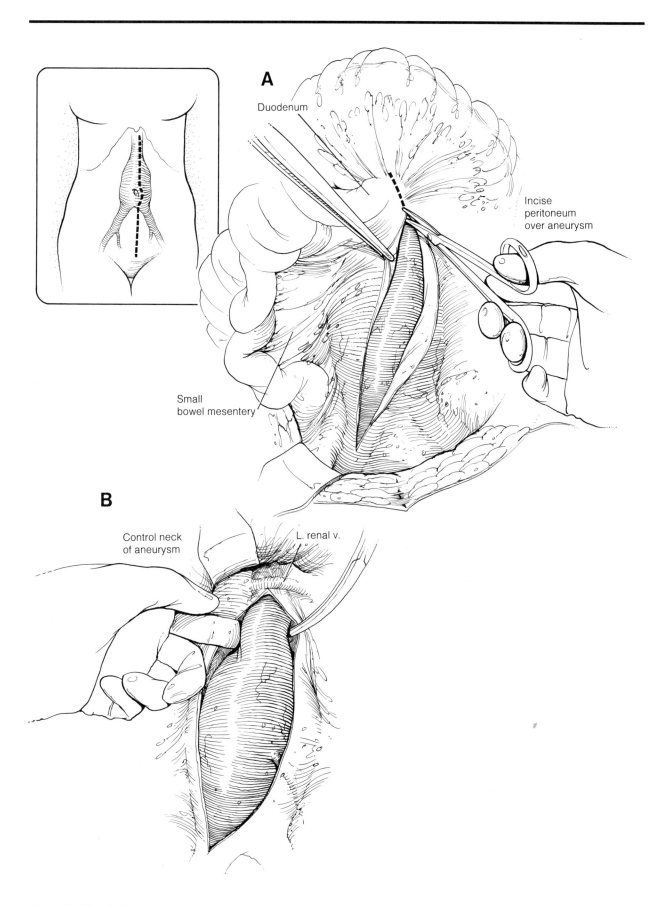

A

Duodenum

Incise
peritoneum
over aneurysm

Small
bowel mesentery

B

Control neck
of aneurysm

L. renal v.

Fig 21–1, C. The inferior mesenteric artery is examined and blood flow velocity evaluated with Doppler ultrasound using a sterile probe to determine patency. If the artery is patent, the Doppler probe is used to evaluate arterial blood flow to the sigmoid colon while temporarily occluding the inferior mesenteric artery. If poor collateral blood flow is detected, the inferior mesenteric artery is reimplanted to the aortic graft during the reconstruction. If collateral blood flow is good, the inferior mesenteric artery is ligated close to the aortic aneurysm. The aorta is occluded proximal to the aneurysm with the "side-winder" aneurysm clamp (Wister modified or DeBakey spoon-shaped aortic clamp). This produces antero-posterior compression of the aorta which allows good visualization of the posterior wall of the aorta for repair. The iliac arteries are occluded bilaterally with 35-degree angle peripheral vascular clamps (DeBakey). An incision is made into the aneurysm after confirmation that there is no longer pulsatile pressure in the aorta. The incision of the aneurysm extends from the neck to the iliac bifurcation.

D. Should any difficulty be encountered in freeing the neck of the aneurysm, the proximal aorta may be controlled and occluded simply by dissecting the sides of the aorta enough to compress it laterally with an aneurysm clamp (DeBakey). The posterior wall of the aorta is less well visualized, but this compromise is advisable in the emergency situation.

E. Contained blood is aspirated from the aneurysm. The use of a cell-saver device is most helpful in conserving blood. The clotted blood and debris are removed from the aneurysm by wiping the wall of the aneurysm with gauze-covered fingers. A plane is developed between the clot and the wall of the aneurysm that enables the operator to remove most of the organized thrombus intact. At times the plane actually includes the intima-media of the aorta as a thromboendarterectomy. Complete removal of this material from the aneurysm makes identification and control of bleeding points much easier and the rest of the repair more tidy.

F. Patent lumbar arteries that are back bleeding are controlled by suture ligature using 2/0 silk. Double loop stitches ("figure of 8") are placed over the orifices of the lumbar arteries. Usually this is sufficient to close the orifice of the vessels and control the bleeding. When this is insufficient, a horizontal mattress stitch around the orifice will actually ligate the vessel and provide the most accurate control of the bleeding point.

A decision is made between using a tube or bifurcated graft for the reconstruction. For aneurysmal deformity that involves only the aorta and spares the iliac arteries, it is possible to insert a simple tubular graft. In these cases, the bifurcation structure will be generally preserved and the iliac arteries will be close to each other with a spur of the aorta between well preserved. It is important to examine the aortic bifurcation for presence of severe calcification or iliac orifice stenosis from within the aorta before making a final decision to use a tube graft. Major abnormality of the aortic bifurcation, atheromatous stenosis of the iliac arteries, or extension of aneurysm into the common iliac arteries dictates the use of a bifurcated prosthesis. The preferred graft is knit Dacron with the interstices of the graft sealed by serum albumin autoclaved into the graft or by commercially prepared grafts sealed with collagen. These grafts have proven to be less permeable than woven Dacron and have the advantage of better long-term tissue incorporation.

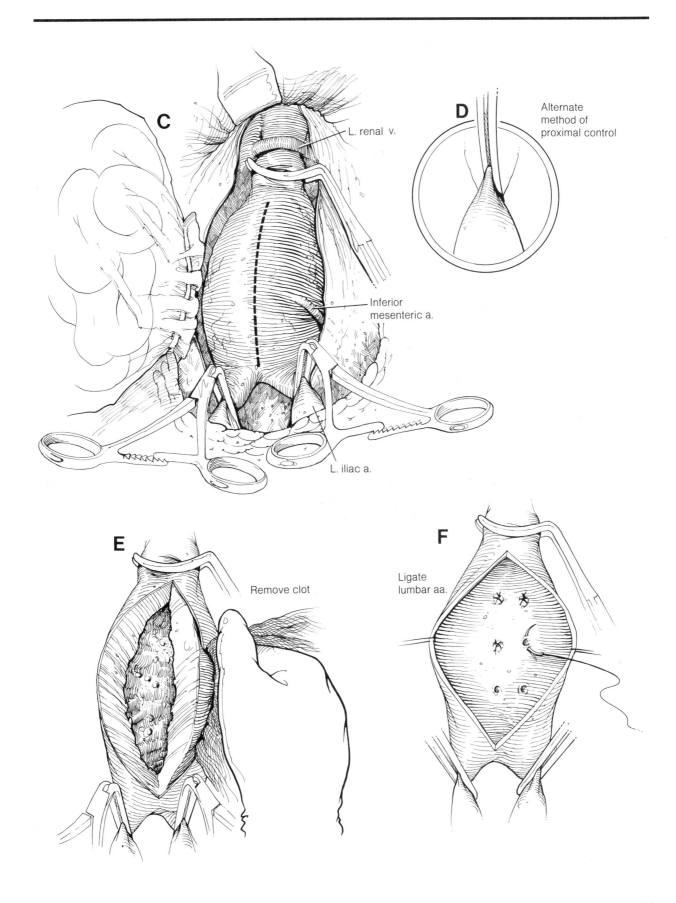

C

L. renal v.

D   Alternate
method of
proximal control

Inferior
mesenteric a.

L. iliac a.

E   Remove clot

F   Ligate
lumbar aa.

Fig 21–1, G.   The aorta is divided proximally at the neck of the aneurysm. This is usually easy to accomplish because there is space between the aorta and the spine. Alternative technique would leave the back wall of the aorta intact and place the graft inside the undivided aorta. Posterior wall security is less with this technique than when the aorta is divided and actual end-to-end anastomosis is constructed.

H.   A 1.5–2.0-cm piece of graft is removed and slipped over the graft to act as a protective cuff. An end-to-end anastomosis of graft to aorta is made using continuous stitches of 3/0 polypropylene suture. The suture loops for the back wall of the anastomosis are placed with the graft held away from the aorta for maximal exposure and accurate stitch placement. The suture line is started through the graft from outside-in and at the left side of the posterior wall of the aorta from inside-out. The stitches are continued across the posterior wall to the outside of the right side of the aorta.

I.   The suture loops for the back wall are pulled up and loop tension adjusted with a nerve hook. The direction of the left side suture and needle are reversed by placement of a mattress stitch so that right-handed stitch placement from inside-out on the aorta may be accomplished working toward the operator.

J.   After the proximal anastomosis is completed, the aortic occlusion clamp is opened slightly to test the integrity of the anastomosis. The cuff is then pulled over the anastomosis to provide extra buttress for protection against false aneurysm formation at the suture line. The distal anastomosis is constructed at the bifurcation of the aorta. The graft is sutured to the undivided aorta from within, taking deep bites of the aortic wall to include the unexposed adventitial layer. The posterior row of sutures is placed with the graft held away from the aorta. The suture loops are tightened up to approximate the graft to the aorta. The cut edge of the aorta anteriorly may be used to incorporate the graft.

K.   The aneurysm wall may be partially resected. Hemostasis must be carefully obtained at the cut edge of the aneurysm. The wall of the aneurysm is closed around the graft by continuous suture. This provides additional protection and isolation of the graft from the abdominal viscera.

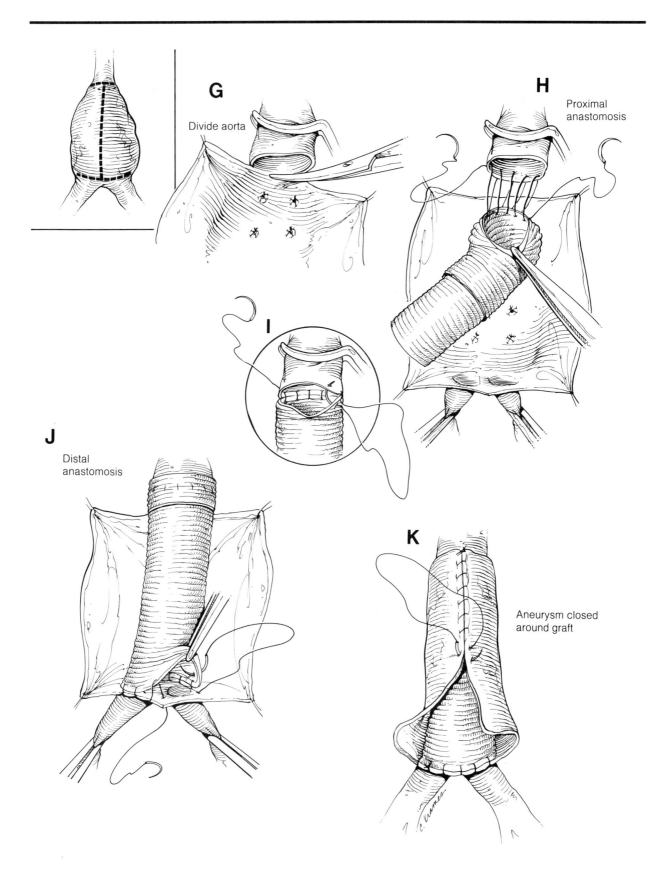

G
Divide aorta

H
Proximal anastomosis

I

J
Distal anastomosis

K
Aneurysm closed around graft

Fig 21–1, L. In cases where the aneurysm involves the proximal iliac arteries, the bifurcation will be destroyed and reconstruction to the individual iliac arteries or even the common femoral arteries required. The incision of the aneurysm should extend into the iliac arteries until near normal diameter vessel is encountered.

L. A bifurcated Darcon graft is employed. The graft is shortened to just above the bifurcation so that sufficient length of the limbs of the graft will allow gentle separation of the limbs to approximate the iliac arteries without kinking. An end-to-end anastomosis of one limb of the graft to the iliac artery is constructed with continuous stitches of 4/0 polypropylene suture. Anastomosis is constructed first to the iliac artery that will be the easiest to perform, so that reperfusion can be rapidly reestablished to one lower extremity. The back wall of the anastomosis is constructed from within the undivided iliac artery taking deep tissue bites to include the adventitia of the artery. The anterior portion of the anastomosis is constructed to the cut edge of the artery. After completion of the first distal iliac artery anastomosis, a soft jaw clamp (Fogarty) is applied to the origin of that graft limb. The aortic occlusion clamp is opened briefly to flush out any residual debris or thrombus, which could have been trapped above the aortic clamp, through the unanastomosed limb of the graft. The soft jaw clamp is moved to occlude the origin of the unanastomosed limb of the graft. The aortic clamp is gradually opened to reperfuse the lower extremity while observing blood pressure and allowing only enough blood flow to enter the leg which will not alter the hemodynamic state significantly. Within a short period, complete reperfusion of the leg is established. The unanastomosed limb of the graft is cleaned out with a suction device. The graft limb is shortened and beveled appropriately to approximate the iliac artery for anastomosis. An end-to-end anastomosis of graft to iliac artery is constructed by continuous suture technique using 4/0 polypropylene. The soft jaw clamp is removed gradually from the graft limb to restore blood flow to the second lower extremity.

M. When the inferior mesenteric artery is found to be necessary for adequate colon blood flow, it is easily reimplanted to the aortic graft. While it is true that this artery can be safely occluded at the aorta in most cases without resultant left colon ischemia, it is also true that reimplantation is not difficult and removes the threat of bowel necrosis. The inferior mesenteric artery is mobilized along with 1-cm button of the surrounding aorta. An appropriate size hole is cut in the graft.

N. The inferior mesenteric artery with its attached button of aorta is anastomosed to the graft by continuous stitch using 4/0 polypropylene.

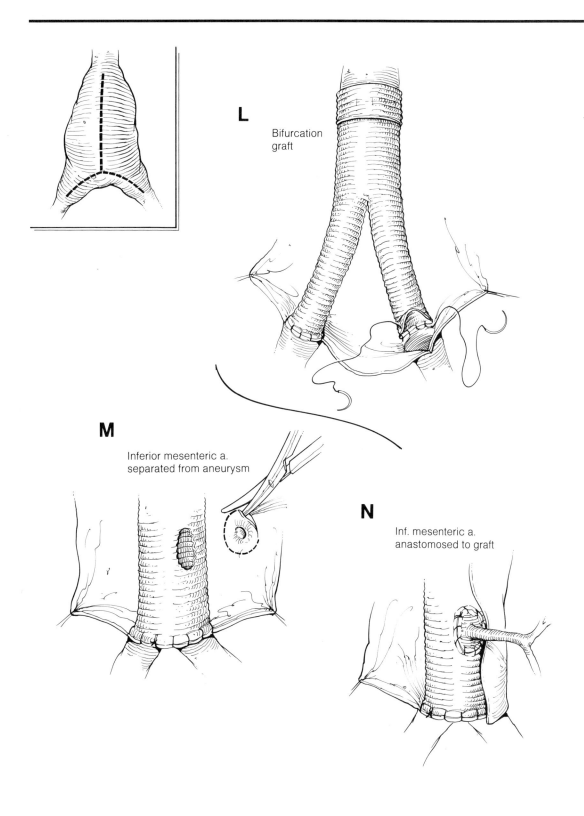

L

Bifurcation
graft

M

Inferior mesenteric a.
separated from aneurysm

N

Inf. mesenteric a.
anastomosed to graft

Ruptured Abdominal Aortic Aneurysm

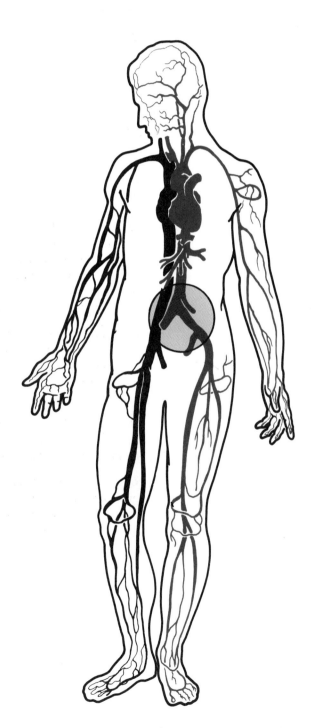

22

Fig 22–1. Operation is an integral part of the resuscitation of a patient with ruptured abdominal aortic aneurysm. Methods and devices for achieving proximal control of the aorta such as vascular occlusion clamps placed on the supraceliac aorta or the thoracic aorta, and balloon catheters inserted retrograde from the femoral artery may be satisfactory in some instances but delay the real resuscitative maneuver of placing the clamp on the aorta at the neck of the aneurysm.

A. There is usually little hemorrhage around the left renal vein so that a small incision of the retroperitoneum at this level will access the aorta without disrupting the retroperitoneal clot.

B. The index and third fingers are gently inserted into the clot which surrounds the aorta and a little space opened on each side of the aorta. The aneurysm is retracted downward and a DeBakey aneurysm clamp closed on the aorta at the neck.

Once the aorta is controlled, resuscitative measures may be continued. The aneurysm is repaired in usual fashion after hemodynamics status stabilize.

Aorta–Inferior Vena Cava Fistula

Aorta–inferior vena cava fistula is the result of abdominal aortic aneurysm which ruptures to the inferior vena cava. The patients often present in circulatory collapse, profound heart failure, and pulmonary edema. The distinguishing feature is the presence of palpable abdominal aortic aneurysm with continuous bruit. At surgery, high venous pressure which declines with aortic occlusion is characteristic. The left to right shunting of blood may cause the inferior vena cava and left renal vein to be distended and have a pink color due to the presence of oxygenated blood. Palpation of a continuous thrill in the aortic aneurysm confirms the diagnosis. The most important resuscitative measure is prompt operation and occlusion of the aorta at the neck of the aneurysm. Control of back bleeding from the vena cava is the unique feature of repair of the aneurysm.

A. The aorta is controlled below the renal arteries at the neck of the aneurysm. No attempt should be made to control the vena cava primarily. Caval pressure will fall with occlusion of the aorta. Heparin (300 units/kg) is administered to raise activated clotting time above 400 seconds. Blood must not clot during salvage and autotransfusion using a cell saver device. The aorta is opened in the usual manner.

B. Suction devices are used to empty the blood contained in the aneurysm. There may be a very large amount of blood flowing back from the vena cava. The fistula, located on the postero-lateral wall of the aneurysm, is controlled by finger occlusion.

C. The fistula is closed beginning at the superior aspect and sewing inferiorly while gradually withdrawing the occluding finger. Deep bites below the finger used to occlude the opening. A large needle on 3/0 polypropylene is used to take deep bites in the tissue until hemostasis is secure. The aneurysm is then repaired in the usual fashion.

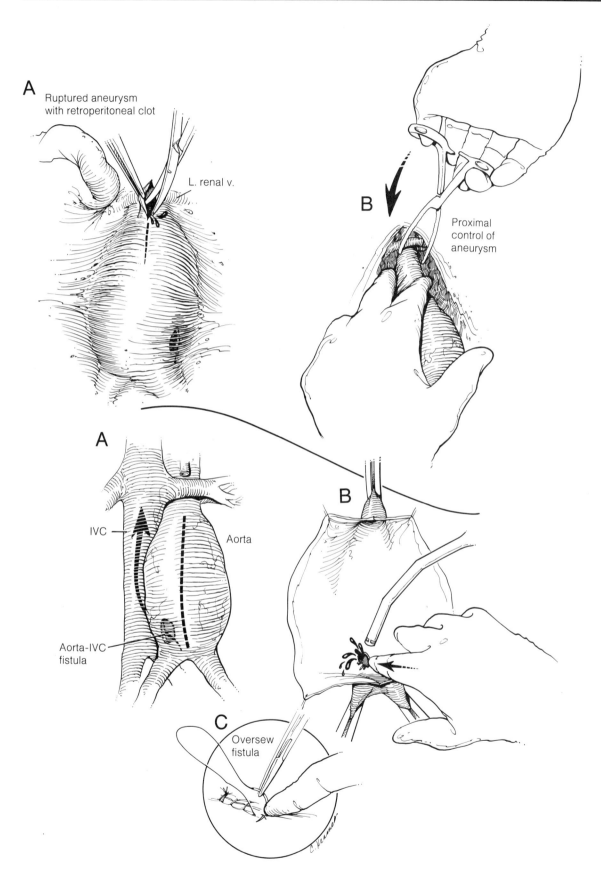

A

Ruptured aneurysm
with retroperitoneal clot

L. renal v.

B

Proximal
control of
aneurysm

A

IVC

Aorta

Aorta-IVC
fistula

B

C

Oversew
fistula

Special Problems Associated With Abdominal Aortic Aneurysm

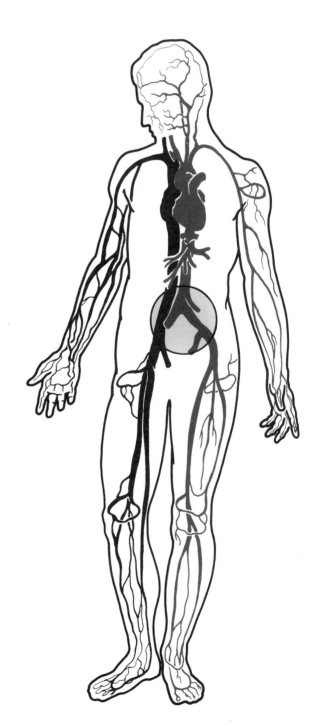

23

Horseshoe Kidney

Fig 23–1. Horseshoe kidney associated with abdominal aortic aneurysm presents the special problem of having renal parenchyma over the bifurcation of the aorta as well as having inferior pole renal arteries originating from the aneurysm. Division of the renal tissue is not required for the repair of the aneurysm. The renal tissue is simply mobilized and retracted so that the aortic branches to the isthmus of the horseshoe kidney can be identified and the prosthetic graft may be worked into the aorta with the kidney minimally disturbed.

A. Dissection is started in the tissue over the aneurysm below the isthmus of the horseshoe kidney. A plane is developed between the kidney and the aorta. Dissection from above the kidney will allow the isthmus to be lifted off the aorta. A retraction tape or Penrose drain is placed around the isthmus of the kidney. Renal arteries originating from the aneurysm are mobilized so that they can be separated from the aneurysm along with a small circular patch of aorta. Proximal and distal control of the aorta is achieved in the usual fashion. The aneurysm is opened in the usual fashion, debris removed, and the lumbar arteries ligated.

B. The aneurysm is repaired using a bifurcated prosthetic graft. The proximal anastomosis is constructed inside the aneurysm or to the divided aorta depending on the circumstances presenting in the individual case. The kidney is retracted inferiorly to gain better exposure of the proximal anastomosis.

C. The limbs of the graft are passed through the space previously created between the aorta and kidney inside the aneurysm. Distal anastomosis of the limbs of the graft to the iliac arteries are constructed in the usual fashion. Accessory renal arteries are reimplanted to an opening in the graft.

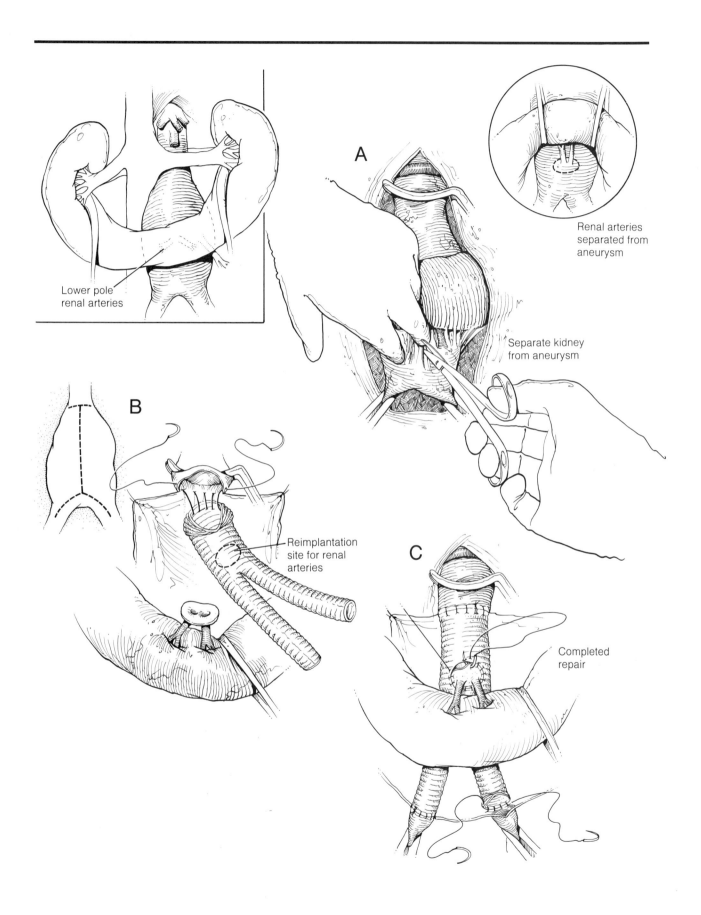

Lower pole
renal arteries

A

Renal arteries
separated from
aneurysm

Separate kidney
from aneurysm

B

Reimplantation
site for renal
arteries

C

Completed
repair

Renal Artery Involvement

Fig 23–2. Juxta-renal artery aneurysm of the abdominal artery presents the problem of managing the origin of the renal arteries. If the aneurysm actually extends above the renal arteries, it will also involve the superior mesenteric artery and the celiac artery so that the aneurysm will have to be managed differently than those aneurysms that are actually juxta-renal and have no neck below the renal arteries. The former type require thoraco-abdominal incision for exposure while the latter may be approached below the transverse mesocolon and pancreas with placement of the aortic occlusion clamp on supra-celiac aorta.

A. The aneurysm is opened right up to the renal arteries. The incision is extended as a "T" at the level of the renal arteries taking care not to enter the renal artery orifices.

B. The posterior row of the anastomosis of aorta to prosthetic graft is performed from within the aorta taking deep bites of tissue to include the aortic adventitia (which is not visualized).

C. The suture line is continuous using 3/0 polypropylene. The stitches are taken in close proximity to the renal arteries, but they are actually below the renal orifices. The anastomosis is completed to the aorta anteriorly.

Accessory Renal Arteries

A. Accessory renal arteries are always reimplanted to the graft when they are encountered during operation for abdominal aortic aneurysm. They can be differentiated from lumbar arteries by their origin from the anterior aspect of the aorta of the aortic aneurysm. The origin of the renal artery and a short segment of the artery are mobilized. The aneurysm is repaired in the usual fashion.

B. A segment of the prosthetic graft that best approximates the original location of the accessory renal artery is isolated and an opening made into it. The accessory renal artery is excised from the aneurysm preserving at least 1 cm diameter of the aortic wall at the origin of the renal artery. The patch of the artery is attached to the opening in the graft by continuous stitch using 4/0 polypropylene suture.

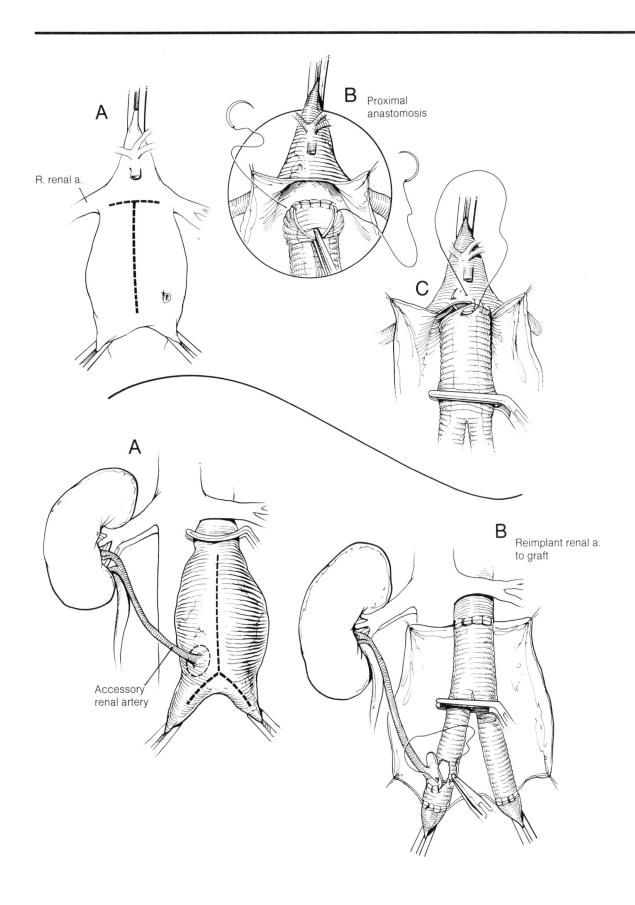

R. renal a.

B Proximal anastomosis

C

Accessory renal artery

B Reimplant renal a. to graft

Aneurysm of Descending Thoracic Aorta

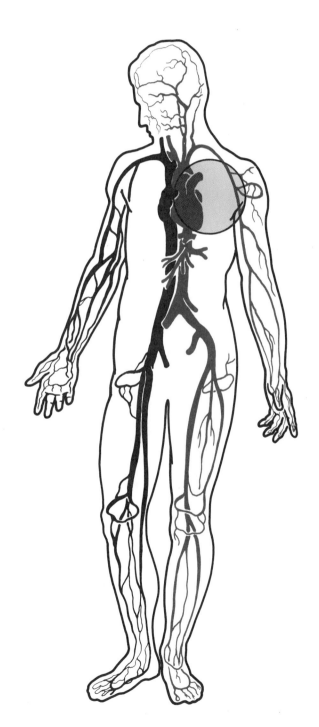

24

Fig 24–1. Aneurysm of the upper portion of the descending thoracic aorta due to atherosclerosis or aortic dissection is approached through a lateral thoracotomy incision. The patient is placed in the right lateral decubitus position (left side up) with the hips and pelvis turned to expose the left groin. A separate incision may be made over the femoral artery to accept the arterial perfusion cannula if the distal thoracic aorta cannot be used.

A. Ascending aorta to descending aorta or femoral artery bypass using a heparin impregnated shunt catheter (Gott shunt) is used to provide blood supply to the lower part of the body and spinal cord as well as control hypertension in the upper compartment. This shunt method offers sufficient control and does not require systemic heparin administration which simplifies hemostasis following repair. Autotransfusion using a cell saver device is a helpful adjuvant to the total care.

B. Proximal control of the aorta should be established as the initial step. When there is sufficient aorta distal to the left subclavian artery, the aorta may be controlled close to the aneurysm. Control of the aortic arch may be necessary to gain sufficient length for repair. The pericardium is opened anterior to the phrenic nerve and retracted to expose the pulmonary artery. An incision is made over the pulmonary artery at the pericardial reflection. The ascending aorta is accessible for cannulation through this incision. Monitoring of the patient consists of pressure lines in left atrium, central systemic vein, and arteries in the upper and lower extremities. Pulmonary arteries and veins are shown divided in the figure for clarity.

The aortic arch is controlled between the left carotid artery and the left subclavian artery by a Robinson catheter. The catheter is attached to the tip of the aneurysm clamp to aid in guiding the clamp around the aortic arch.

C. The aorta distal to the aneurysm is controlled close to the aneurysm, leaving sufficient aorta available for the repair. The aorta is occluded proximal and distal to the aneurysm with aneurysm clamps. The subclavian artery is occluded separately. The shunt is opened to control blood pressure in the upper compartment and to assure cerebral and spinal cord blood flow without excessive afterload of the left ventricle. The aneurysm is incised through its length. Side extensions of the incision define the limits of resection of the aneurysm. The contained blood, clot, and debris are removed.

D. Intercostal arteries are ligated from within the aneurysm while deciding if reimplantation of some of the intercostal arteries should be done. The aneurysm may be repaired from within, or the aorta may be divided for open end-to-end anastomosis.

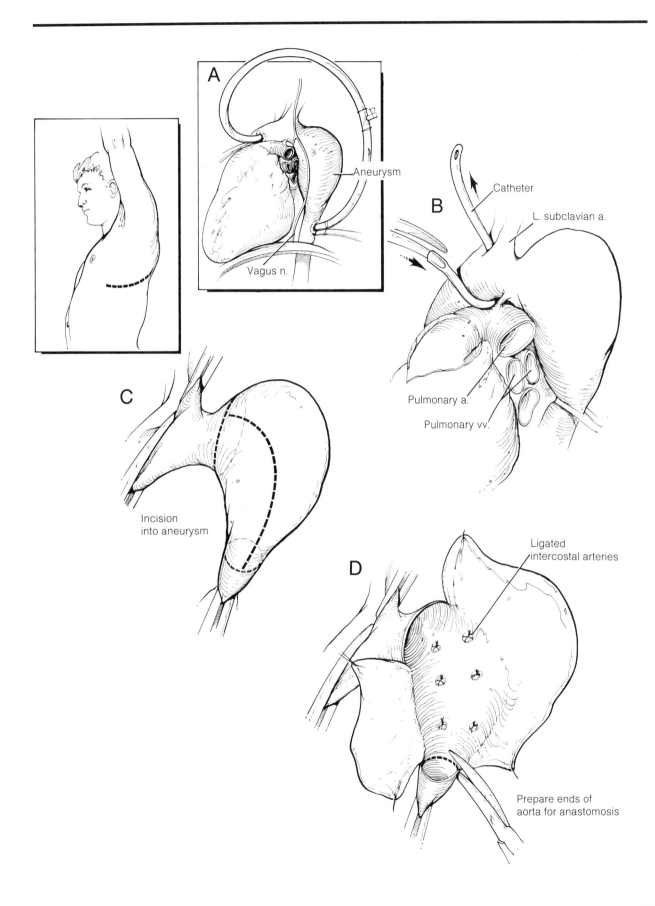

A

Aneurysm

Vagus n.

B

Catheter

L. subclavian a.

Pulmonary a.

Pulmonary vv.

C

Incision
into aneurysm

D

Ligated
intercostal arteries

Prepare ends of
aorta for anastomosis

Fig 24–1, E. An appropriate size tubular Dacron graft is chosen for the reconstruction. Double velour knitted or woven grafts that have been impregnated with concentrated albumin and autoclaved for three minutes are favored. An end-to-end anastomosis of graft to proximal aorta is constructed by continuous stitches of 3/0 polypropylene. Several suture loops are placed posteriorly prior to pulling up the suture to approximate the graft to the aorta. Deep bites must be taken so that the full thickness of the aorta is included.

F. The anastomosis is completed anteriorly by transition from within the aorta to full inside-out technique. The needle arc must be controlled so that needle perforations in the tissue do not form slits.

G. In cases of aortic dissection, it is necessary to prepare the end of the aorta prior to anastomosis. While it is possible to simply reconstruct the aorta to the graft, it is in practice easier and better to reconstruct the aorta separately and then restore continuity by the graft. Strips of Teflon felt are placed inside the aorta against the intima of the "true" lumen and on the outside of the aorta against the adventitia. A continuous mattress stitch is used to approximate the strips of Teflon felt to the aorta while at the same time obliterating the "false" channel caused by the dissection of the intima-media.

H. End-to-end anastomosis of graft to the divided aorta has some advantage in that the full thickness of the posterior wall is always included but accomplished at the expense of more dissection of the aorta to free up the back wall sufficiently. A collar or the graft may be cut from the end and slipped onto the graft prior to anastomosis. End-to-end anastomosis is accomplished by continuous suture technique using 3/0 polypropylene.

I. The completed aortic reconstruction is reinforced at the suture lines by covering with a Dacron collar and closure of the aneurysm around the graft.

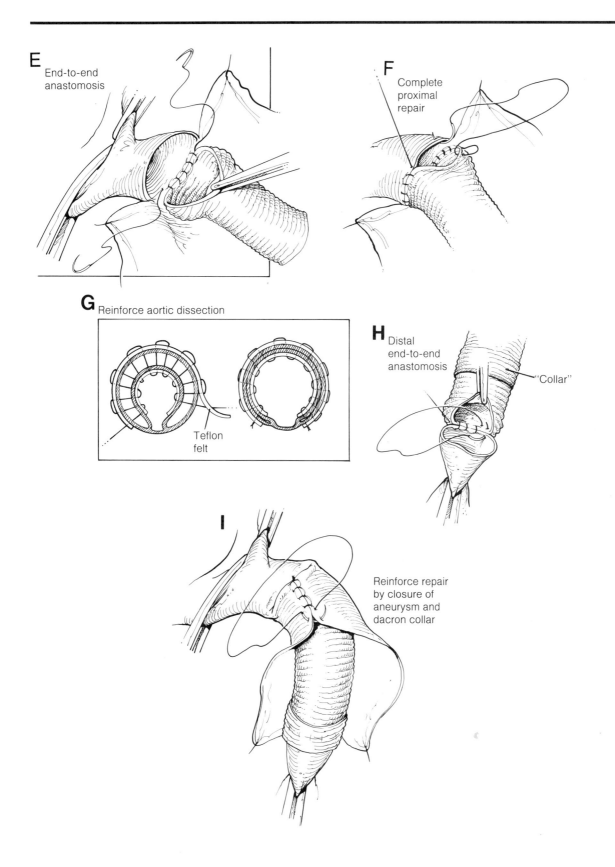

E End-to-end anastomosis

F Complete proximal repair

G Reinforce aortic dissection

Teflon felt

H Distal end-to-end anastomosis

"Collar"

I

Reinforce repair by closure of aneurysm and dacron collar

Thoraco-abdominal Aortic Aneurysm

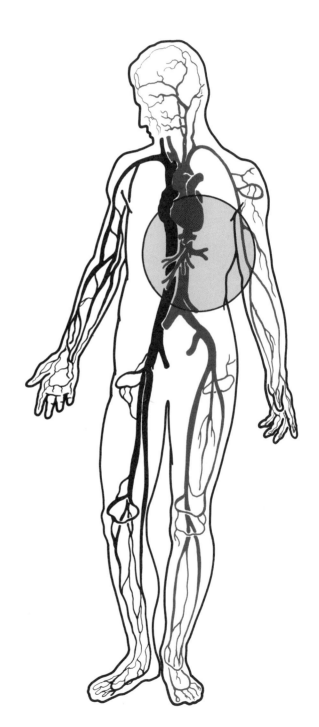

25

Fig 25–1. Aneurysm of the aorta extending from the thoracic aorta into the abdominal aorta is amenable to operative treatment. The operation is complex and associated with significant potential for morbidity because the blood supply to the spinal cord and the kidneys is involved, placing these organs at risk for ischemic injury.

The patient is positioned about 60 degrees left side up. The operating table may later be rotated to reduce the degree of side up positioning. A thoraco-abdominal incision is used. The thoracic portion of the incision is placed on the chest wall to provide access to the fifth intercostal space. The incision crosses the costal margin to the midline of the upper abdomen and continues in the midline to a point below the umbilicus.

A.   The periosteum of the fifth rib is elevated from its inferior aspect. The left pleural space is entered through the bed of the nonresected fifth rib. The lung is retracted superiorly to expose the diaphragm. The ribs are separated with a self-retaining retractor. The abdominal portion of the incision is through the linea alba to the preperitoneal space but does not enter the peritoneal cavity. Dissection is started in the preperitoneal space to free the peritoneum from the inferior surface of the diaphragm. The diaphragm is perforated in the costophrenic sulcus anteriorly. The costal cartilages are divided without entry to the peritoneal cavity.

B.   The chest retractor is spread more widely. The peritoneum is dissected from the inferior surface of the diaphragm more completely so that the stomach, spleen, and left kidney are mobilized out of the left upper quadrant of the abdomen and retracted medially and anteriorly. The dissection is taken down to the aorta. This prepares the diaphragm for incision without entering the peritoneal cavity. Real effort should be made to keep the peritoneum intact as the abdominal contents are well contained and much easier to control.

C.   The diaphragm is incised with scissors or cautery blade in radial fashion down to and through the aortic hiatus. The retractor is more widely separated providing complete exposure of the thoraco-abdominal aorta. Further dissection and mobilization of the peritoneum from the surface of the aorta inferiorly may be required. The lung is retracted superiorly to gain access to the superior margin of the aneurysm.

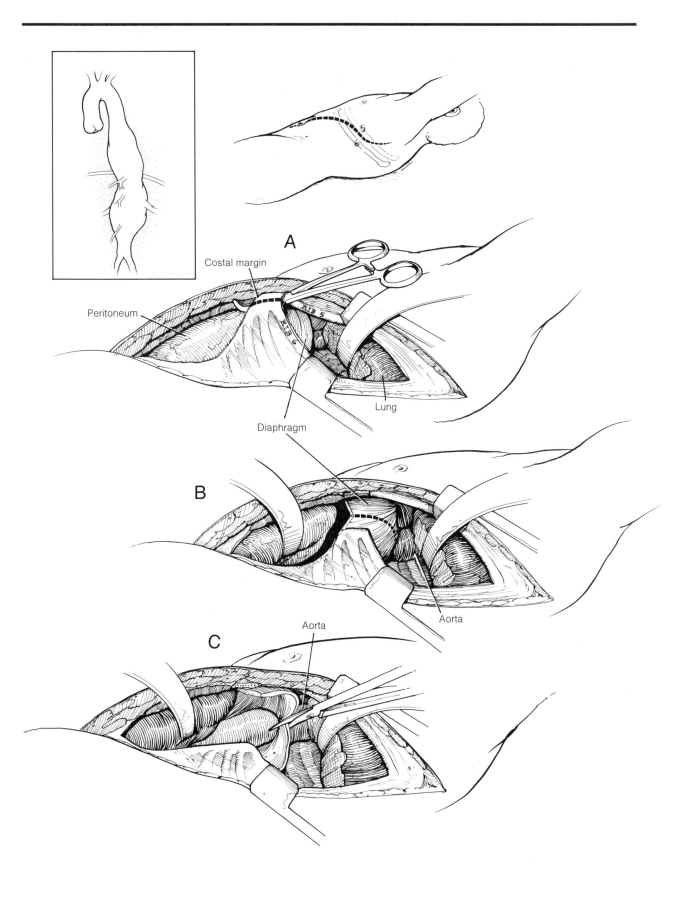

A

Costal margin

Peritoneum

RIB 5

RIB 6

Diaphragm

Lung

B

Diaphragm

Aorta

C

Aorta

Fig 25–1, D. The aorta is controlled proximal and distal to the aneurysm. Only the minimal dissection of the vessel to obtain control is done. The aortic branches are not dissected at all. The illustration shows the visceral vessels as if freed up from the surrounding tissues. This has been done for clarity of illustration, but in practice, these vessels are not seen at all. The vessels are buried in the fat and connective tissue anterior to the aorta. Only the lateral wall of the aorta is exposed. Administration of heparin is controversial. Certainly anticoagulation makes a safer operation in terms of clot formation in the visceral or lower extremity arteries. On the other hand, anticoagulation may present more difficulty when it comes to obtaining hemostasis. Generally, we would advise the use of heparin. In all cases, a cell saver device should be employed. The aorta is occluded proximal and distal to the aneurysm, placing the vascular clamps as close to the aneurysm as possible while maintaining adequate margin for control and anastomosis. The aortic branches are not clamped and are simply allowed to back bleed to the aortic lumen. If this back bleeding seems excessive and provides difficulty obtaining adequate exposure, balloon catheters may be inserted for intraluminal control. The aorta is opened through the length of the aneurysm. A "T"-shaped incision defines proximal and distal limits of the aneurysm resection.

E. Thrombus and other debris contained within the aneurysm are removed by fingers covered with gauze. The debris should be removed as completely as possible. Retraction stitches are placed on the edges of the aneurysm for exposure.

F. The orifices of the visceral arteries are identified from within the aorta. Large intercostal arteries at the level of the diaphragm may be preserved. Lumbar branches are occluded by suture ligature. The aorta is divided proximal to the aneurysm.

G. A double velour knitted Dacron prosthesis rendered impervious by soaking in albumin and passing through the autoclave is used for the reconstruction. A cuff of the graft is fashioned to reinforce the proximal anastomosis. An end-to-end anastomosis of the graft to the aorta is constructed using 3/0 polypropylene suture. Suture loops for the entire back row are placed with the graft held away from the aorta. The suture loops are pulled up to approximate graft to aorta. The anterior row of sutures are then placed to complete the anastomosis.

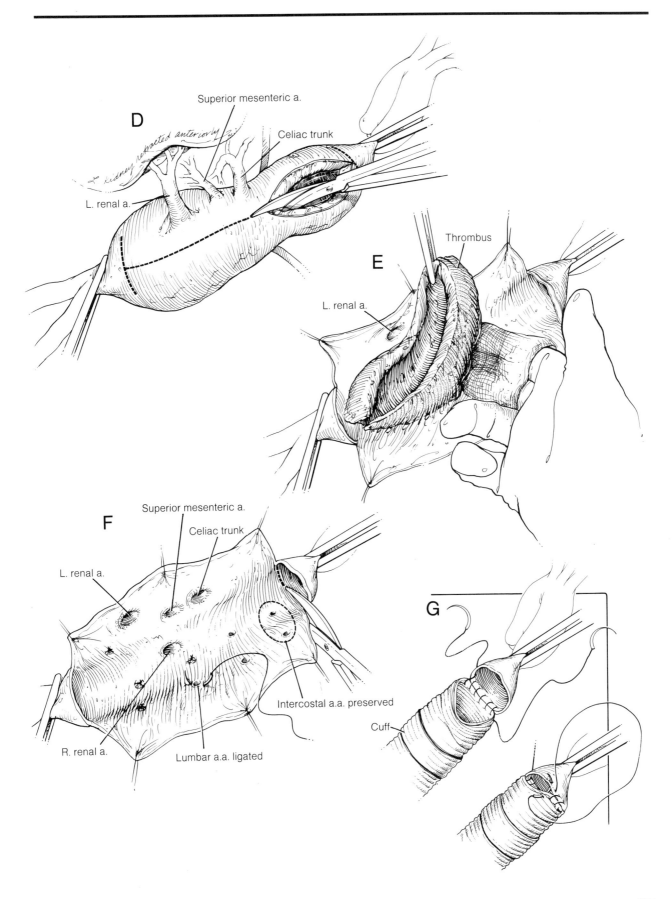

D

L. kidney retracted anteriorly

Superior mesenteric a.

Celiac trunk

L. renal a.

E

Thrombus

L. renal a.

F

Superior mesenteric a.

Celiac trunk

L. renal a.

Intercostal a.a. preserved

R. renal a.

Lumbar a.a. ligated

G

Cuff

Fig 25–1, H. The proximal anastomosis is tested by temporarily opening the aortic occlusion clamp. After determining the suture line is adequate, the cuff is slipped over the anastomosis. If there is a large pair of patent intercostal arteries about the level of the diaphragm, these may be reimplanted to the graft. A round opening is made into the graft. The graft is simply sewn to the aortic wall around the intercostal artery orifices. Substantial tissue bites are taken for maximum suture line security using continuous stitches of 3/0 polypropylene.

I. The visceral arteries are anastomosed to the graft. An opening to the graft is formed that is large enough to encompass the origins of the celiac artery, superior mesenteric artery, and the right renal artery. Care must be taken to consider the anterior rotation of the visceral artery orifices in planning the graft openings. This usually means making the opening more toward the left side of the graft than might be apparent at first glance. The left renal artery is generally anastomosed separately to prevent kinking at the anastomosis. The anastomosis is constructed by continuous suture technique using 3/0 polypropylene suture. Deep tissue bites are taken for security of the suture line.

J. The left renal artery is anastomosed to a separate opening in the graft by similar technique. The position of the anastomosis should be planned carefully, taking into account the amount of anterior rotation and displacement of the left renal artery produced by the mobilization of the left kidney.

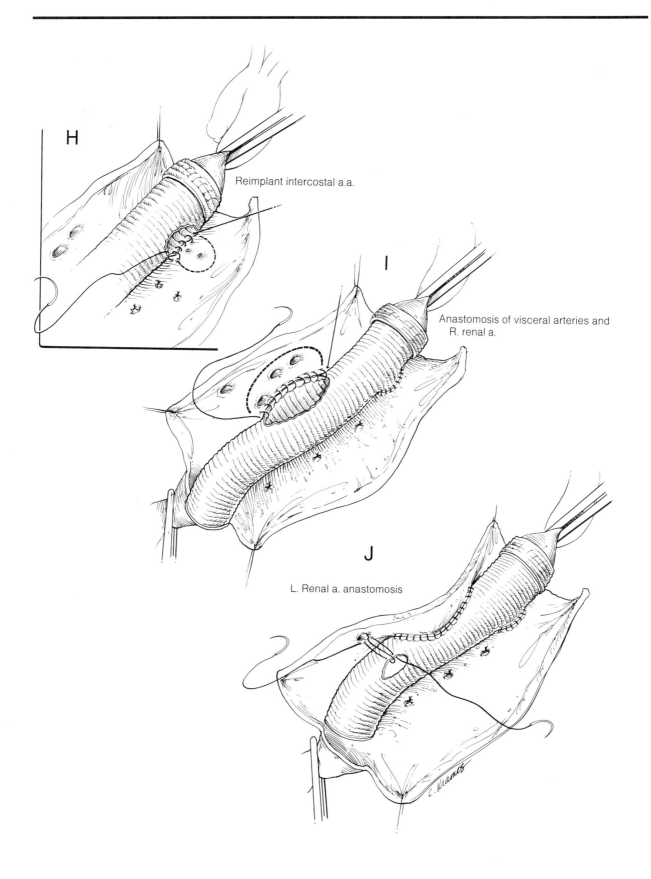

H   Reimplant intercostal a.a.

I   Anastomosis of visceral arteries and R. renal a.

J   L. Renal a. anastomosis

Fig 25–1, K. There are some variations to be considered for the visceral artery anastomoses. Variation I might be considered when renal artery position seems to dictate a better fit of the graft to the arteries if separate anastomoses are made to the right and left renal arteries. Variation II would be one in which all four visceral arteries are anastomosed separately. The latter variation probably would be performed rarely.

L. The distal anastomosis of graft to the aorta is constructed in end-to-end fashion. The back row of the anastomosis is to the intact wall of the aorta so that deep tissue bites must be taken to be sure that the suture engages the aortic adventitia posteriorly. For situations in which the aneurysm extends into the common iliac arteries, it is necessary to employ a bifurcated graft. The limbs of the graft are anastomosed to the iliac arteries in modified end-to-end fashion, keeping the posterior wall of the iliac arteries intact. The aneurysm is closed around the graft at the completion of all the anastomoses and after suture line hemostasis is secured.

K

Variation I

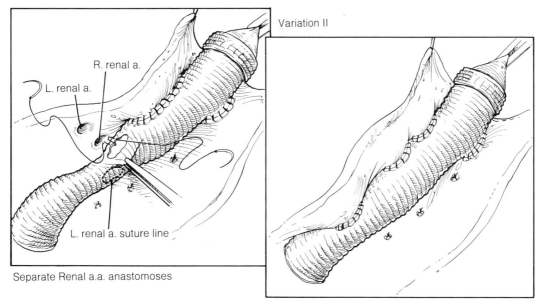

L. renal a.

R. renal a.

L. renal a. suture line

Separate Renal a.a. anastomoses

Variation II

Individual arterial anastomoses

Complete distal anastomosis

L

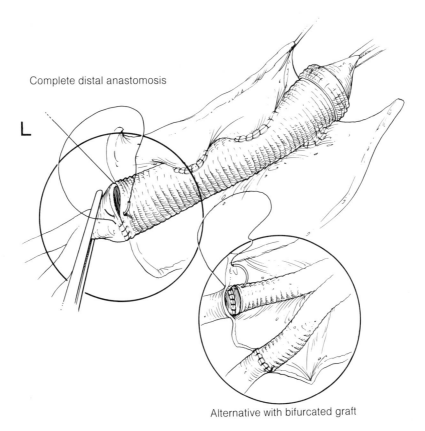

Alternative with bifurcated graft

Renal Artery
Revascularization

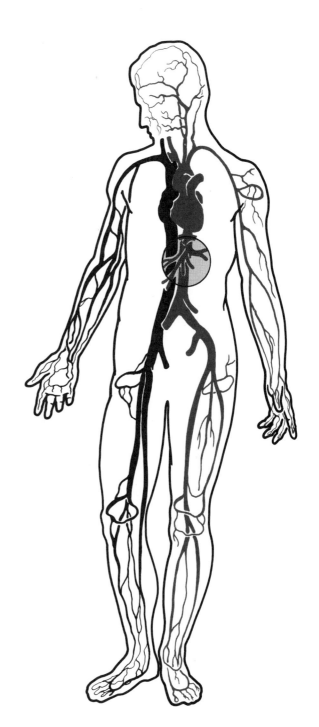

26

Fig 26–1. Revascularization of a stenosed renal artery is performed for the treatment of arterial hypertension and in selected cases without hypertension as an associated procedure when treating abdominal aortic lesions.

The renal arteries are usually approached via a midline abdominal incision that extends from the xyphoid process of the sternum to the symphysis pubis. A self-retaining ring retractor enhances exposure of the renal arteries.

A. An incision is made in the peritoneum to the left of the fourth portion of the duodenum over the abdominal aorta. The small intestine is placed outside the peritoneal cavity in a Lahey bag and retracted to the right. The aorta is dissected from the retroperitoneal tissues from the level of the inferior mesenteric artery to a level above the crossing point of the left renal vein. This vein must be completely mobilized so that it can be retracted away to expose the renal arteries that lie behind it. During the dissection of the left renal vein, its tributaries should be identified. The left adrenal vein joins the left renal vein on its superior aspect. The gonadal vein joins the left vein on its inferior aspect. The inferior vena cava is exposed only as required to obtain adequate mobilization of the renal veins and exposure of the renal arteries.

B. Exposure of the left renal artery is obtained by ligation of the left adrenal vein and the left gonadal vein. This allows complete mobilization of the left renal vein. The vein is retracted superiorly and somewhat to the right to allow access to the left renal artery that lies behind.

C. The right renal artery at its origin is exposed by thorough mobilization of the left renal vein and the inferior vena cava. Retraction of the junction of the left renal vein with the inferior vena cava to the right and superiorly exposes the origin of the left renal artery.

D. The distal portion of the right renal artery is exposed by thorough mobilization of the right renal vein after ligation of its branches. The right renal vein is retracted superiorly to gain access to the distal right renal artery which lies behind.

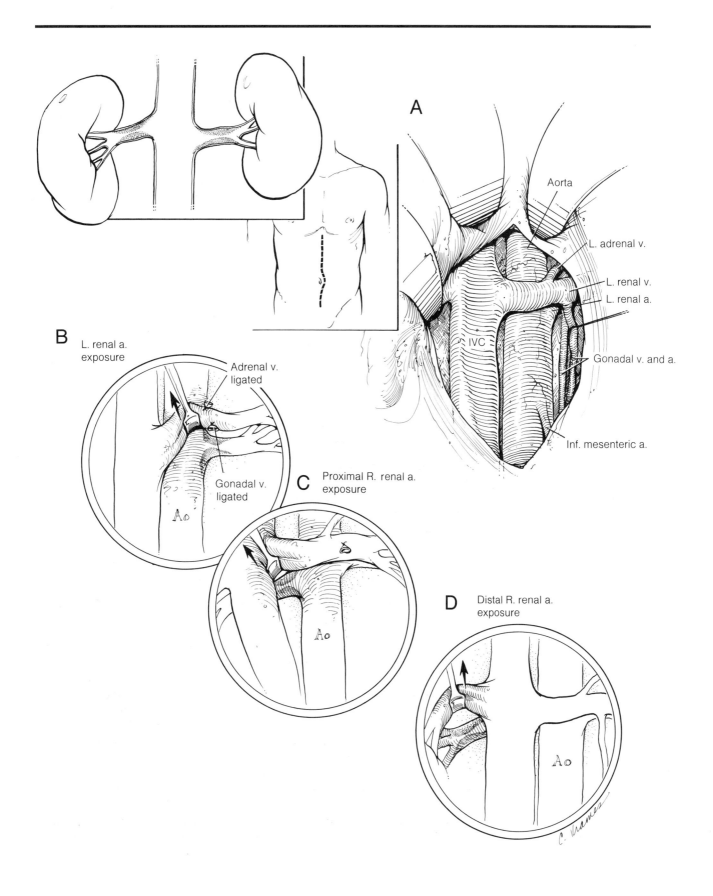

A

Aorta

L. adrenal v.

L. renal v.

L. renal a.

Gonadal v. and a.

IVC

Inf. mesenteric a.

B L. renal a.
exposure

Adrenal v.
ligated

Gonadal v.
ligated

Ao

C Proximal R. renal a.
exposure

Ao

D Distal R. renal a.
exposure

Ao

Renal Artery Revascularization

Aorto-renal Artery Bypass

A. Bypass of the renal artery is performed using the saphenous vein as the bypass conduit in most cases. Prosthetic material (PTFE-Gortex or Dacron) may be used in selected cases but is not as reliable as autogenous bypass grafts. The saphenous vein is removed from the thigh by usual techniques. A portion of the aorta located between the crosspoint of the left renal vein and the origin of the inferior mesenteric artery is isolated by curved vascular clamp (Lambert-Kay). This clamp may be placed to only partially occlude the aorta, but in practice, it nearly always totally obstructs the aorta when enough aorta is isolated to make anastomosis easy. A circular opening is made into the aorta using an aortic punch (Karp or coronary) about 4 to 5 mm in diameter depending on the size of the vein graft. An end-to-side anastomosis of the vein graft to the aorta is constructed by continuous stitches of 5/0 polypropylene. The proximal portion of the anastomosis off the aorta to the "heel" of the beveled vein graft is performed with the vein graft held apart from the aorta as the first five suture loops are placed. This provides accurate approximation of the most important portion of the anastomosis. The remainder of the anastomosis is constructed by continuous stitch. Alternatively, the anastomosis to the aorta may be performed as a completion step of the procedure after the vein graft to the renal artery is performed.

B. The renal vein is retracted to expose the renal artery. The renal artery is ligated proximally and divided distal to the atherosclerotic disease. A slight bevel is made when dividing the artery to obtain an increased circumference for anastomosis.

C. Fibromuscular dysplasia stenoses in the renal artery in the hilum of the kidney beyond the branching point are treated by catheter balloon dilation.

D. The saphenous vein graft is shortened appropriately to accurately bridge between the aorta and the cut end of the renal artery. Excess length may kink the graft. An end-to-end anastomosis of vein bypass graft to the renal artery is constructed with 5/0 or 6/0 polypropylene suture. A very small needle may be desirable if the area of exposure is small. A "stay" stitch at one end of the anastomosis is used to stretch out the vein graft as the continuous suture line is started at the opposite end. The sutures must be accurately placed and the curved needle carefully withdrawn so as not to produce the slightest injury to the renal artery. Optical magnification is used.

E. The posterior row of the anastomosis is performed first and the sutures placed anteriorly to complete the repair.

A'. An alternative method of creating the bypass is to perform an end-to-side anastomosis of the vein bypass graft to the renal artery. A curved vascular clamp is used to isolate a portion of the renal artery. A longitudinal incision is made into an area of the renal artery which is free of atheromatous disease. The vein graft is shortened to approximate the renal artery by dividing it with an appropriate bevel. The anastomosis is constructed by continuous stitches of 5/0 to 6/0 polypropylene. The initial stitch is placed from the intimal surface to the outside of the "heel" of the vein graft. Using the opposite needle of the double needle suture, the second stitch is placed through the proximal angle of the renal arteriotomy from the intimal surface to the outside. This needle is then brought from the outside into the lumen of the vein graft. The inferior portion of the anastomosis can then be constructed by placing the stitches from the intimal surface of the renal artery, directly through the wall of the artery to the adjacent vein graft. The superior portion of the anastomosis is constructed to complete the repair.

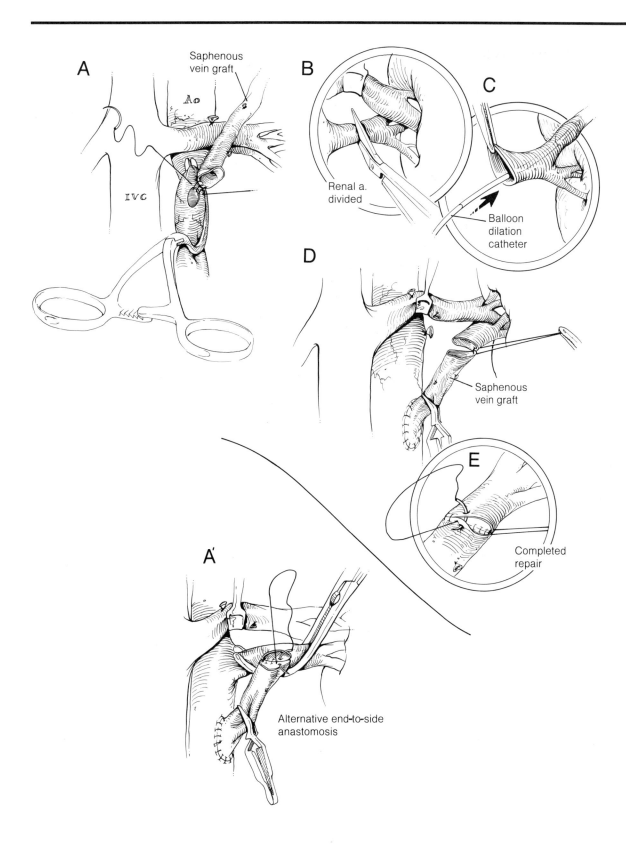

A

Saphenous vein graft

Ao

IVC

B

Renal a. divided

C

Balloon dilation catheter

D

Saphenous vein graft

E

Completed repair

A'

Alternative end-to-side anastomosis

Reimplantation of Renal Artery

Fig 26–3. Reimplantation technique may be considered for stenosis of the renal artery which is located in the origin of the renal artery and does not extend into the artery. Thorough mobilization of the renal artery is required to obtain enough length for this procedure.

A. The origin of the renal artery is isolated along with a generous portion of the aorta below using a curved vascular clamp. The renal artery is occluded distally by vascular clamp. The renal artery is ligated and divided as close to the aorta as possible through artery that is uninvolved in the atheromatous process. The renal artery will be reimplanted to a normal site on the aorta below the original site.

B. A circular opening is made into the aorta using the Karp aortic punch or a disposable coronary aortic punch. An end-to-side anastomosis of the renal artery to the aorta is constructed with 5/0 polypropylene. The anastomosis is set up so that the needle will pass from the intimal surface of the renal artery to the aorta. This is accomplished by taking the initial stitch from the intimal surface of the aorta to the outside at the superior aspect of the aortotomy. The needle at the opposite end of the double needle suture is then passed from the intimal surface of the renal artery to the outside. This needle is continued and brought from the outside back into the aorta. The suture line may then proceed from the intimal surface of the renal artery to the adjacent aorta.

C. The repair is completed by continuing the suture line along the anterior aspect of the aortotomy.

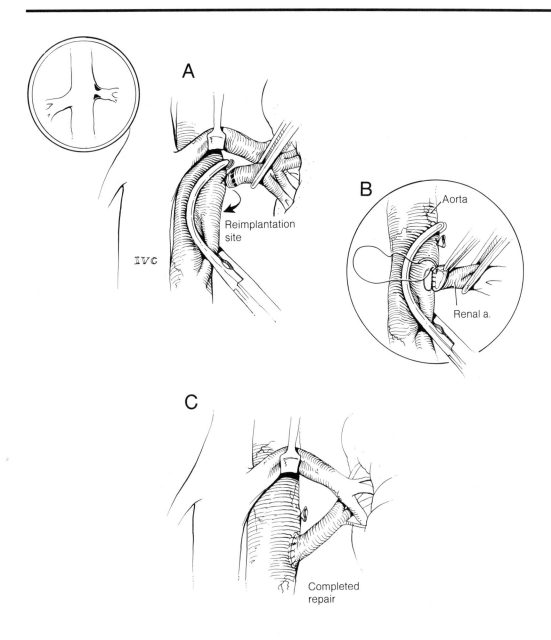

A

IVC

Reimplantation
site

B

Aorta

Renal a.

C

Completed
repair

Aorto-renal Endarterectomy

Fig 26–4. Aorto-renal endarterectomy may be performed for disease of the origin of the renal arteries. The atherosclerotic stenosis should be short and limited to the orifice of the renal arteries. In practice, it is most applicable in combination with aortic graft operations. In those cases, the infra-renal aorta is divided so that opening the aorta anteriorly for a short distance (3 cm) greatly improves renal artery orifice exposure. This is easily closed and the aortic occlusion clamp moved below the origin of the renal arteries for completion of the aortic reconstruction. The operation is more difficult to perform than bypass or reimplantation procedures because more extensive exposure and mobilization of the aorta and the renal arteries are required. The problem of achieving an accurate endpoint for the endarterectomy is similar to endarterectomy procedures performed in other arteries except that the exposure is more difficult.

A. The aorta and renal arteries are completely mobilized. The inferior vena cava is mobilized and cleared away from the right renal artery. The left renal vein is thoroughly mobilized and retracted superiorly so that the aorta may be occluded proximal to the renal arteries with a vascular clamp. The aorta is also occluded below the renal arteries. The renal arteries are occluded by vascular clamp as far lateral to the aorta as is permissible by the exposure. A longitudinal arteriotomy is made at the center of the aorta opposite the renal artery orifices.

B. A plane is started in the media of the aorta to dissect the atheromatous plaque away from the media-adventia layer of the aorta. The dissection plane is extended into the renal arteries. The endpoint is achieved as the dissection of the plaque blends to more normal intima. The dissector breaks through the intima and separates the plaque from the artery.

C. The opposite renal artery is treated similarly with dissection and removal of the atheromatous plaque. The end of the plaque must appear tapered. The plaque must be removed cleanly or else the renal artery will have to be opened and the endpoint assured. If the endpoint does not taper properly, the renal artery can be transected distally at a point where the intima is normal and intact. The proximal renal artery is cleaned out by endarterectomy and the renal artery reanastomosed in end-to-end fashion using interrupted stitches of 6/0 polypropylene.

D. The arteriotomy is closed by direct suture with polypropylene to complete the repair.

A'. The alternate approach is through a transverse arteriotomy. The advantage of this incision is better visualization of the endpoint of the plaque within the renal artery. The disadvantage is the requirement of direct closure of the renal artery rather than simply closing the aorta.

B'. The dissection plane is started in the aorta and extended into the renal arteries.

C'. The endpoint is developed under direct vision. The plaque must be carefully tapered.

D'. The arteriotomy is closed by continuous suture with special care at each end of the incision not to narrow the renal artery.

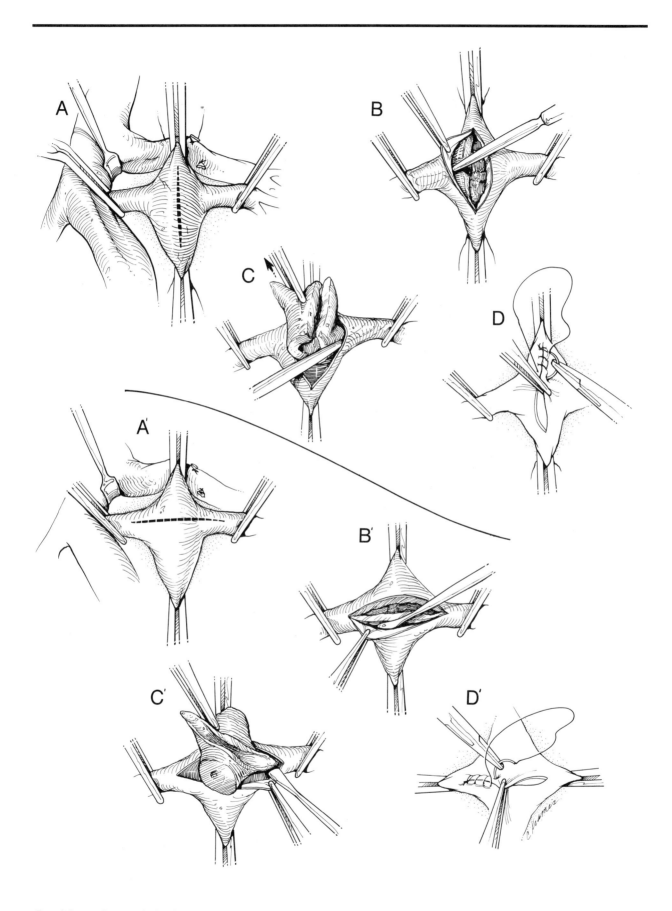

Spleno-renal Artery Bypass

Fig 26–5. The splenic artery may be used as a bypass conduit to the left renal artery. It is especially useful for reoperation in patients with late aorto-renal artery vein bypass graft stenosis. The proximal renal artery and aorta need not be exposed in this operation. The splenic artery is large and will carry sufficient blood flow to relieve renal artery stenosis. Unfortunately, the artery is tortuous and brittle, making it somewhat difficult to use. The exposure is even more extensive than for other renal artery procedures that may be exposed working beneath the transverse mesocolon. Mobilization of the splenic artery carries the small but definite risk of inducing pancreatitis. The spleen, however, need not be removed as it will survive nicely on its other blood supply from the short gastric arteries.

A. The gastroepiploic arteries are divided and the pancreas exposed through the lesser sac. The stomach is retracted superiorly, the transverse colon retracted inferiorly. The splenic artery is mobilized from the superior margin of the pancreas. Branch vessels to the pancreas are ligated and divided. The splenic artery is ligated and divided at the hilum of the spleen. The artery is mobilized medially to the celiac artery. The left renal artery and vein are dissected from beneath the tail of the pancreas into the hilum of the kidney.

B. The splenic artery is passed through a tunnel created posterior to the pancreas. The pancreas is retracted superiorly to expose the renal blood supply. The renal vein is retracted inferiorly after ligating its branches. An end-to-side anastomosis of the splenic artery to the left renal artery is constructed with 5/0 to 6/0 polypropylene suture using continuous stitches. The anastomosis is started at the "heel" of the somewhat beveled end of the splenic artery. Fine suture loops are placed around the "heel" and the end of the longitudinal arteriotomy in the left renal artery. The two arteries are approximated and the anastomosis continued along the posterior edge of the arteriotomy. The anastomosis is completed anteriorly.

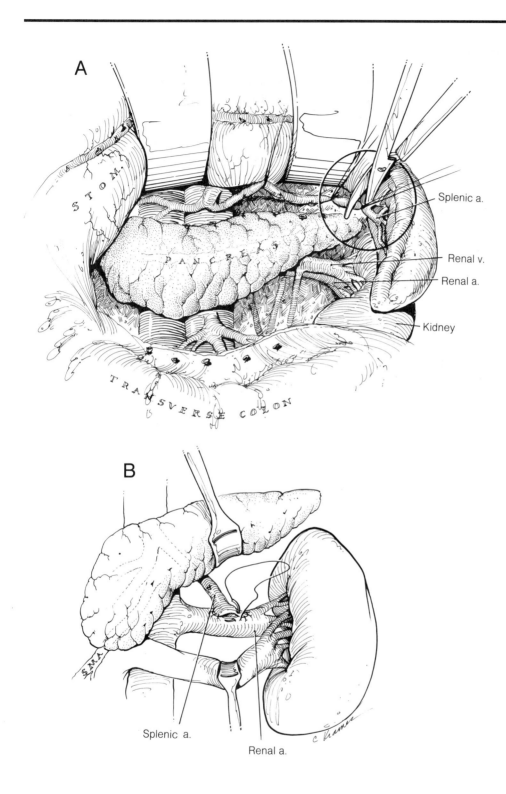

A

Splenic a.

Renal v.

Renal a.

Kidney

B

S.M.A.

Splenic a.

Renal a.

Renal Artery Embolectomy

Fig 26–6,A. Obstruction of the renal artery caused by embolic material is relieved by removal of the embolus by balloon catheter. The aorta is mobilized above and below the affected renal artery. Vascular clamps are applied to the aorta to isolate the renal artery. A small arteriotomy is made on the aorta opposite the renal artery. The embolectomy catheter is passed from the aorta to the renal artery. The balloon is inflated and the catheter withdrawn from the aorta. The embolus is displaced from the renal artery and retrieved from the aorta.

Renal Artery Aneurysmectomy

A'. The aneurysm of the renal artery is exposed by thorough mobilization of the renal artery and vein. The vein is retracted superiorly. The renal artery is ligated proximal to the aneurysm. The renal artery is divided proximal and distal to the aneurysm. The aneurysm is excised. A short segment of saphenous vein is removed from the thigh and anastomosed to the aorta below the origin of the renal artery. The end of the vein graft is beveled to approximate the angle of bevel created on the renal artery when it was divided.

B'. An end-to-end anastomosis of the vein graft to the renal artery is constructed with 5/0 to 6/0 polypropylene using techniques described for renal artery bypass.

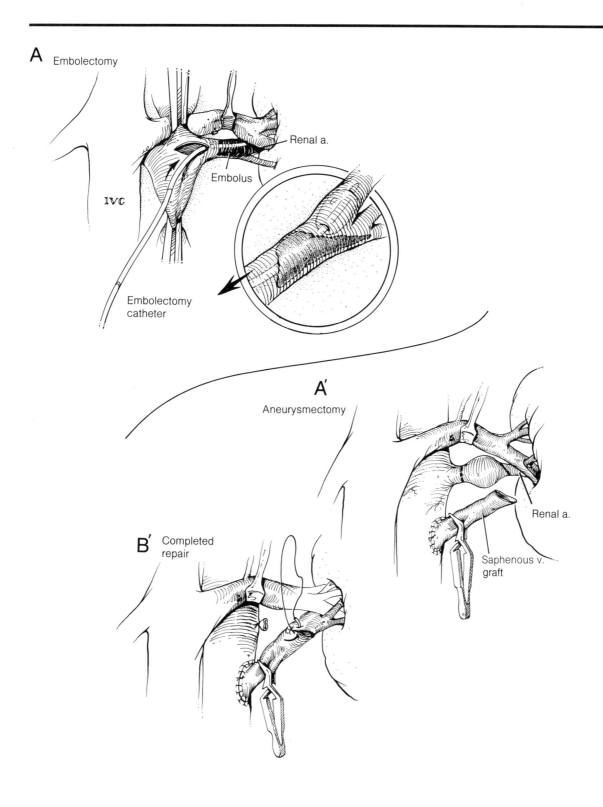

A Embolectomy

Renal a.

Embolus

IVC

Embolectomy
catheter

A'
Aneurysmectomy

Renal a.

Saphenous v.
graft

B' Completed
repair

Superior Mesenteric and Celiac Artery Revascularization

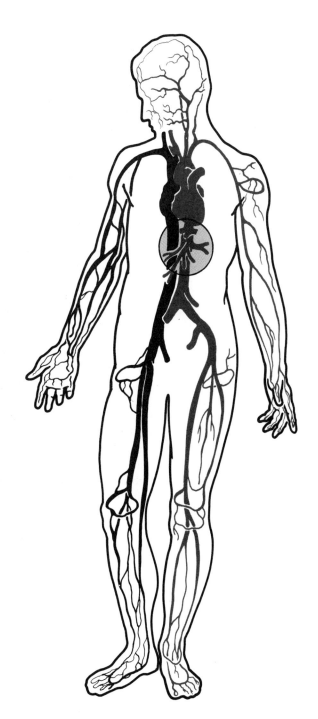

27

Superior Mesenteric Artery Embolectomy

Fig 27–1, A.   There are two common acute disease processes that affect blood flow through the superior mesenteric artery: (1) atherosclerotic obstruction of the origin of the artery with stenosis and acute occlusion by thrombosis; and (2) embolus to the artery. Embolic disease usually affects the artery more distally with the embolic material lodging distal to the origin of the middle colic artery so that colon blood supply is spared for the most part. Differential diagnosis is based on the different angiographic pattern with each of these conditions.

_B._   A midline incision is made in the abdomen extending from the xyphoid process to the pubis. The abdominal contents are explored and potential for restoring bowel viability determined. The diagnosis of embolus to the superior mesenteric artery is made by absence of pulsation in the arteries supplying the jejunum and ileum while pulsation is present in the middle colic artery. The omentum and transverse colon are placed on moist packs outside the body on the anterior chest wall. The small bowel is placed into a plastic bowel bag (Lahey) and taken outside the peritoneal cavity to the right side. An incision is made in the peritoneum over the aorta at the ligament of Treitz.

_C._   The aorta is mobilized from just below the left renal vein to the origin of the inferior mesenteric artery in case bypass graft is required to revascularize the superior mesenteric artery. A second peritoneal incision is made in the base of the small bowel mesentery to expose the superior mesenteric artery as it emerges from below the inferior margin of the pancreas and crosses anterior to the third portion of the duodenum. Sufficient length of the superior mesenteric artery is mobilized to control it and allow for arteriotomy. Vessel loops are placed around the main artery. Small branches need not be controlled because there will be little back bleeding.

_D._   A vascular clamp is placed on the artery proximally. A transverse arteriotomy is performed. A balloon embolectomy catheter is used to extract the embolus from the artery. A 3F or 4F catheter is usually about the right size.

_E._   The proximal artery is flushed out by removing the vascular clamp temporarily. The arteriotomy is closed by continuous stitch using 5/0 polypropylene. After reestablishing superior mesenteric artery blood flow, the quality of the arterial blood flow velocity is determined by Doppler ultrasound using a sterile probe. Papaverine, 30 mg, is injected directly into the superior mesenteric artery through a 25-gauge needle to help relieve spasm of the distal arterial bed. The bowel is inspected visually for viability and the Doppler probe used to assess blood flow in the distal arterial arcades as well as along the bowel mesentery. Before closure of the abdomen, a decision should be made regarding the need for a ''second look'' exploratory laparotomy at 24 hours after operation.

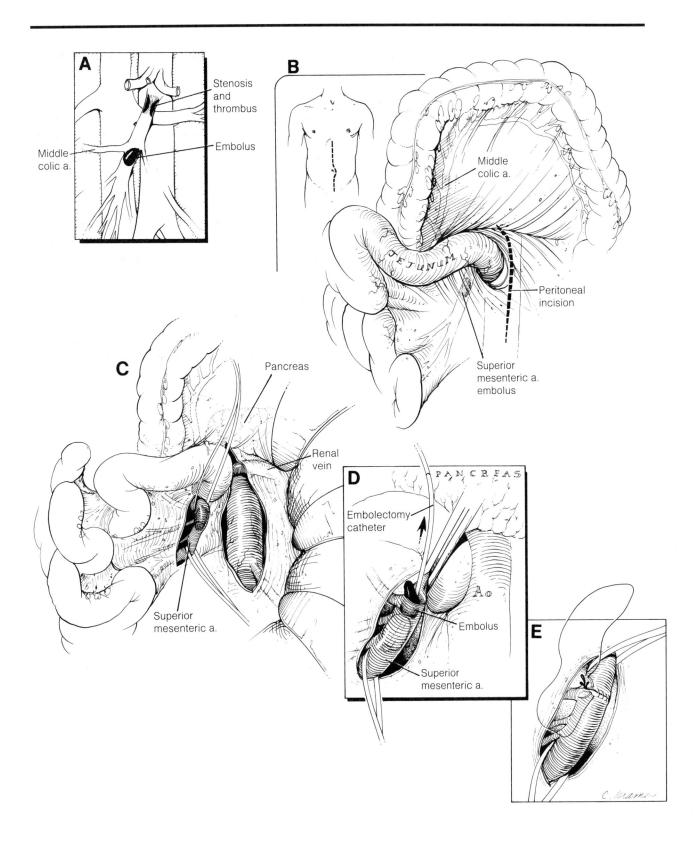

A

Middle colic a.

Stenosis and thrombus

Embolus

B

Middle colic a.

JEJUNUM

Peritoneal incision

Superior mesenteric a. embolus

C

Pancreas

Renal vein

Superior mesenteric a.

D

PANCREAS

Embolectomy catheter

Ao

Embolus

Superior mesenteric a.

E

Superior Mesenteric Artery Thrombectomy With Aorta to SMA Saphenous Vein Bypass Graft

Fig 27–2, A. Proximal atherosclerotic lesion in the superior mesenteric artery may occlude the artery by associated thrombosis. In this situation, pulsation will be absent in the middle colic artery. A longitudinal arteriotomy is made in the superior mesenteric artery; the thrombus, which may be present in the artery distal to the primary obstruction, is extracted using forceps and a balloon embolectomy catheter. A segment of the infra-renal aorta is isolated using a curved vascular clamp (Lambert-Kay). A circular arteriotomy is made in the aorta using a punch device.

B. A short segment of saphenous vein is removed from the groin. An end-to-side anastomosis of the vein graft to the arteriotomy in the superior mesenteric artery is performed. The initial five suture loops are placed at the heel of the graft prior to approximating the graft to the artery.

C. The vein graft is then anastomosed in end-to-side fashion to the aorta. Continuous stitch of 4/0 or 5/0 polypropylene is used for both anastomoses.

D. The operative approach to revascularize the superior mesenteric artery is, therefore, through the peritoneal cavity below the transverse mesocolon into the base of the small bowel mesentery.

SUPERIOR MESENTERIC A. THROMBECTOMY
WITH AORTA-SMA VEIN GRAFT

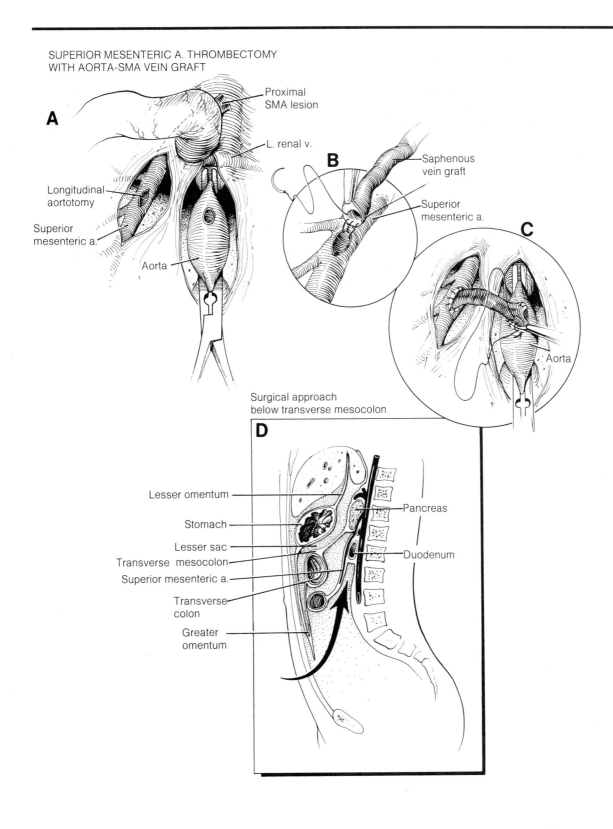

A

Proximal
SMA lesion

L. renal v.

Longitudinal
aortotomy

Superior
mesenteric a.

Aorta

B

Saphenous
vein graft

Superior
mesenteric a.

C

Aorta

Surgical approach
below transverse mesocolon

D

Lesser omentum

Stomach

Lesser sac

Transverse mesocolon

Superior mesenteric a.

Transverse
colon

Greater
omentum

Pancreas

Duodenum

Celiac Axis Revascularization

Fig 27–3, A.   The celiac axis is exposed in the lesser peritoneal sac. A midline abdominal incision is made and the stomach and intestines packed inferiorly. The lesser omentum is opened through an avascular area above the lesser curvature of the stomach to enter the lesser sac. The peritoneum above the pancreas is incised to expose the celiac axis. The muscle fibers of the aortic crus of the diaphram may be incised to enhance exposure of the origin of the artery. The artery is dissected from the dense neurolymphatic tissue of the celiac plexis to control the origin and the branches.

B.   The aorta is mobilized alongside the origin of the artery to allow placement of a curved vascular clamp to isolate that portion of the aorta containing the celiac artery.

C.   When the stenosis involves only a short segment at the origin of the celiac artery, the artery may be reimplanted to the aorta. The artery is divided distal to the obstructing disease and the proximal end oversewn. An arteriotomy is made with a punch device more distal on the aorta. An end-to-side anastomosis of the celiac artery to the aorta is constructed by continuous suture.

D.   If the celiac artery is short and reimplantation seems awkward, a short segment of saphenous vein may be interposed to gain sufficient length to reattach the artery to the aorta.

E.   When the atherosclerotic disease extends the length of the celiac artery to the origin of the branches, a useful alternative is bypass from aorta to the hepatic artery using saphenous vein graft.

F.   Thus, the operative approach to the celiac axis is via the lesser peritoneal sac through the lesser omentum in the upper abdomen.

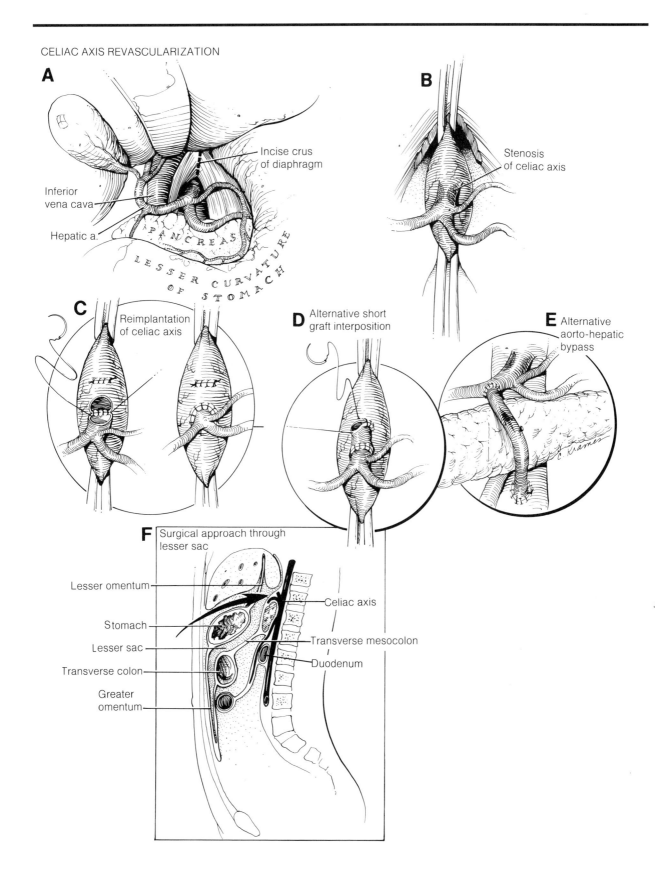

A

Incise crus of diaphragm

Inferior vena cava

Hepatic a.

PANCREAS

LESSER CURVATURE OF STOMACH

B

Stenosis of celiac axis

C

Reimplantation of celiac axis

D Alternative short graft interposition

E Alternative aorto-hepatic bypass

C. Krames

F Surgical approach through lesser sac

Lesser omentum

Stomach

Lesser sac

Transverse colon

Greater omentum

Celiac axis

Transverse mesocolon

Duodenum

Chronic Mesenteric Artery Occlusion

Fig 27–4. Chronic obstruction of the mesenteric artery with abdominal pain syndromes or malnourishment is nearly always associated with significant obstruction of the celiac axis. All of the blood supply to the intestine is involved. Revascularization usually means a combined approach to both the superior mesenteric artery and the celiac axis. This is accomplished by using bypass grafts of the greater saphenous vein taken from the groin.

A. The hepatic artery is mobilized working through the lesser peritoneal sac.

B. The superior mesenteric artery and the upper portion of the infra-renal aorta are mobilized working below the transverse mesocolon through the peritoneal cavity. A curved vascular clamp (Lambert-Kay or Cooley) is used to isolate a segment of the aorta. Two aortotomies are made using a punch device. A longitudinal arteriotomy is made in an isolated portion of the superior mesenteric artery.

C. A segment of saphenous vein graft is placed between the aorta and the superior mesenteric artery. A second vein graft is attached to the aorta for bypass to the hepatic artery.

D. The hepatic vein graft is taken through the transverse mesocolon to the lesser sac, where it lies posterior to the duodenum and anterior to the pancreas.

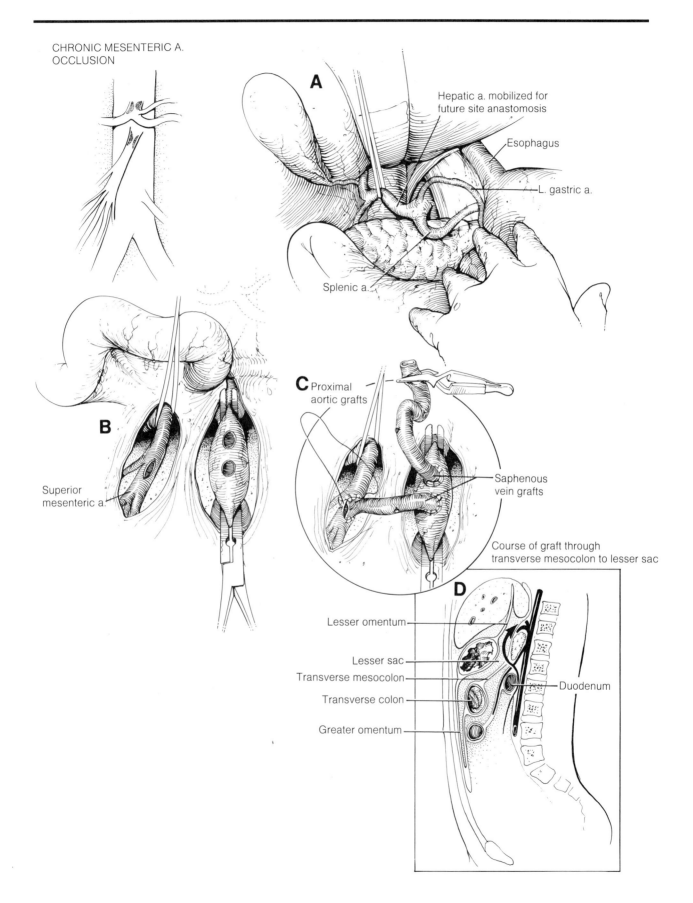

CHRONIC MESENTERIC A.
OCCLUSION

A

Hepatic a. mobilized for
future site anastomosis

Esophagus

L. gastric a.

Splenic a.

B

Superior
mesenteric a.

C Proximal
aortic grafts

Saphenous
vein grafts

Course of graft through
transverse mesocolon to lesser sac

D

Lesser omentum

Lesser sac

Transverse mesocolon

Transverse colon

Greater omentum

Duodenum

Fig 27–4, E.   An opening is made in the transverse mesocolon to the left of the fourth portion of the duodenum. A tunnel is created through the mesocolon anterior to the pancreas. The lesser sac is entered as the superior leaf of the peritoneum of the transverse mesocolon is perforated. The vein graft is taken through this tunnel to approximate the mobilized hepatic artery.

F.   An arteriotomy is made in the isolated hepatic artery. An end-to-side anastomosis of the saphenous vein graft to the hepatic artery is constructed. The completed repair provides blood flow to both the superior mesenteric artery and the celiac axis via bypass grafts from the aorta.

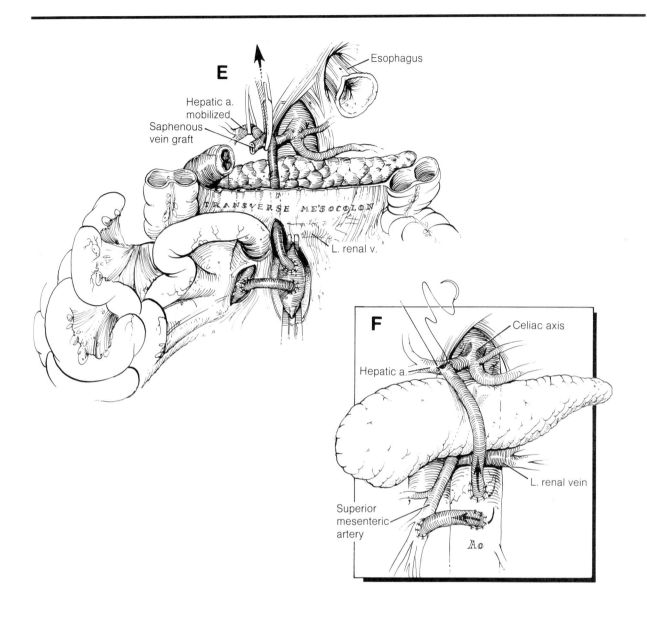

28

Aneurysm of Other Visceral Arteries

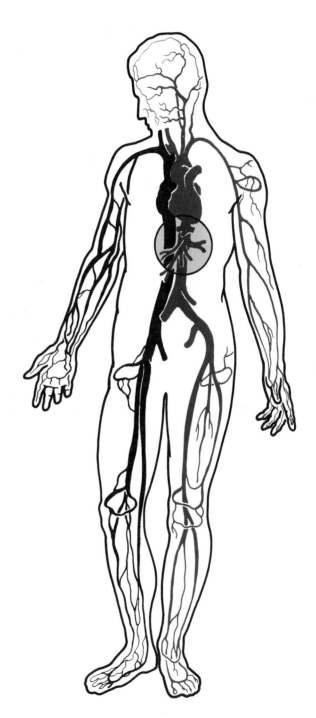

Fig 28–1. Apart from revascularization of the blood supply to the small intestine, the essential pathology of the visceral arteries is aneurysm. Prevention of rupture is the main indication for operative intervention in patients with aneurysm of visceral arteries.

Splenic Artery Aneurysm

A. Aneurysm of the splenic artery may be located at any point in its course from the celiac artery to the hilum of the spleen. Dual blood supply to the spleen via the short gastric arteries from the left gastroepiploic artery makes it possible to remove a splenic artery aneurysm without excision of the spleen.

B. The aneurysm is exposed at the superior margin of the pancreas. The splenic artery proximal and distal to the aneurysm is ligated and the aneurysm excised. The spleen is left in situ with blood flow to the hilum via the short gastric arteries.

Common Hepatic Artery Aneurysm

A. Aneurysm of the common hepatic artery is approached via the lesser peritoneal sac. The aneurysm is isolated and the hepatic artery controlled proximal and distal to the aneurysm. The aneurysm is excised.

B. The hepatic artery cannot be mobilized sufficiently to bring the ends together after removal of the aneurysm. A segment of saphenous vein is removed from the leg and used to reconstruct the hepatic artery. An end-to-end interposition graft is constructed.

Celiac Artery Aneurysm

A. Aneurysm of the celiac artery is approached through the lesser peritoneal sac. The aneurysm is mobilized. The left gastric artery must be sacrificed in order to remove the aneurysm and restore blood flow to the critical hepatic artery.

B. Mobilization of the hepatic and splenic artery often provides sufficient length to allow end-to-end anastomosis of the celiac arterial stump to the confluence of hepatic and splenic artery.

C. The completed repair restores blood flow to the hepatic and splenic artery with the left gastric artery ligated.

D. Should mobilization of the hepatic and splenic artery be insufficient to allow end-to-end anastomosis, the alternative of a saphenous vein interposition graft is employed.

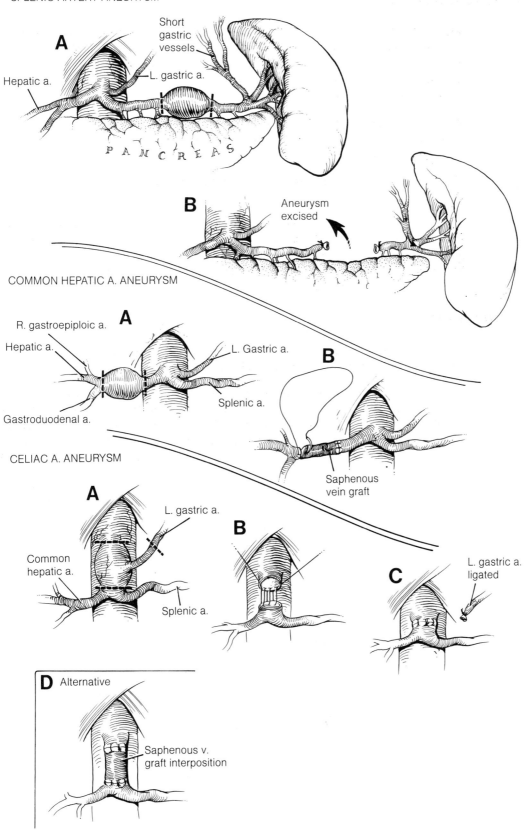

SPLENIC ARTERY ANEURYSM

A Short gastric vessels

Hepatic a.

L. gastric a.

P A N C R E A S

B Aneurysm excised

COMMON HEPATIC A. ANEURYSM

R. gastroepiploic a.

Hepatic a.

A

L. Gastric a.

B

Splenic a.

Gastroduodenal a.

Saphenous vein graft

CELIAC A. ANEURYSM

A

L. gastric a.

Common hepatic a.

B

C L. gastric a. ligated

Splenic a.

D Alternative

Saphenous v. graft interposition

Superior Mesenteric Artery Aneurysm

Fig 28-2. Aneurysm of the superior mesenteric artery is usually located near its origin from the aorta. These aneurysms are commonly mycotic in origin. This should be carefully considered in making intraoperative decisions regarding ligation and resection without reconstruction, provided collateral flow is satisfactory. Culture for bacteria and fungi should be done routinely.

A. The aneurysm is approached through incision in the peritoneum at the base of the small bowel mesentery over the superior mesenteric artery. A second incision is made in the peritoneum over the aorta.

B. The superior mesenteric artery is controlled proximal and distal to the aneurysm. The aneurysm is excised.

C. The proximal end of the superior mesenteric artery is oversewn. Blood supply to the small bowel is restored by saphenous vein graft from the aorta to the distal superior mesenteric artery. The vein graft is taken from separate incision in the groin. An end-to-side anastomosis of graft to the aorta and an end-to-end anastomosis of graft to superior mesenteric artery is constructed.

Inferior Mesenteric Artery Aneurysm

A. The aneurysm of the inferior mesenteric artery is mobilized along with the left colic artery and the superior hemorrhoidal artery. The aneurysm is excised.

B. It is usually possible to reimplant the bifurcation of the inferior mesenteric artery onto the aorta at a point lower than the origin of the inferior mesenteric artery. A circular opening is made into the aorta with the Karp aortic punch at a point that approximates the distal remnant of the inferior mesenteric artery. An end-to-side reimplantation anastomosis is constructed to restore blood supply to the left colon, sigmoid, and rectum.

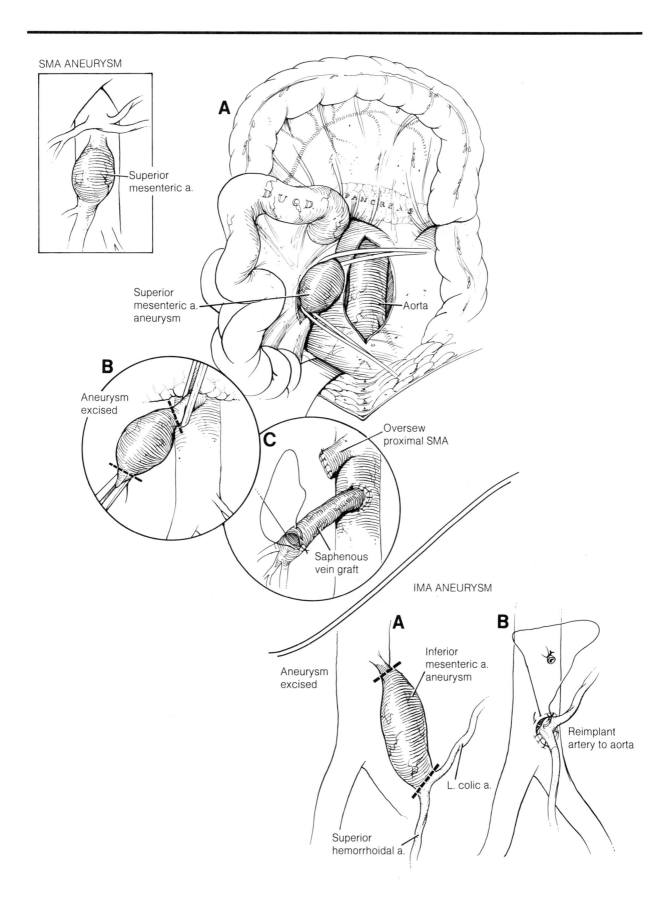

SMA ANEURYSM

A

Superior mesenteric a.

Superior mesenteric a. aneurysm

Aorta

B

Aneurysm excised

C

Oversew proximal SMA

Saphenous vein graft

IMA ANEURYSM

A

Aneurysm excised

Inferior mesenteric a. aneurysm

L. colic a.

Superior hemorrhoidal a.

B

Reimplant artery to aorta

Arterial Embolectomy

29

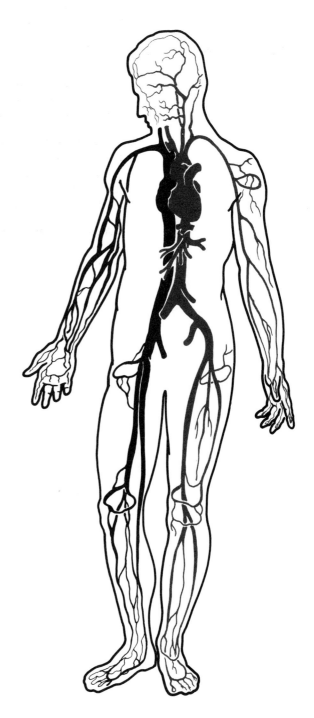

Fig 29–1. The common source of arterial emboli is mural thrombus from the endocardial surface of the heart. The left atrial appendage in patients with atrial fibrillation or the scarred endocardial surface of the ventricle after myocardial infarction are the usual sites for thrombus that may break loose and migrate through the arteries to some peripheral location. Arterial emboli tend to lodge at arterial bifurcation points. The most common sites for emboli to locate are the bifurcation of the carotid or brachial arteries in the upper compartment. In the lower part of the body, the bifurcation of the aorta, femoral or popliteal arteries, or the renal arteries are the usual sites of involvement with arterial embolus. Embolic material removed from the arteries should always be examined histologically. While most emboli will be simply organized thrombus, occasional embolus of tumor (myxoma) or septic vegetation will be discovered.

Aortic Bifurcation Embolectomy

Embolus to the aortic bifurcation is approached through bilateral incisions over the femoral artery in the groin. It would be extremely unusual for abdominal incision to be required although it is best to have the abdomen prepared into the operative field.

A. The common femoral, profunda femoris, and superficial femoral arteries are dissected and controlled. Vascular clamps are applied to these arteries for hemostasis. A longitudinal (not transverse) incision is made into the common femoral artery. A longitudinal incision is preferred because the arteriotomy may be used for aorto-femoral artery bypass should embolectomy fail to open the aorta.

B. An arterial embolectomy catheter is inserted into the common femoral artery. The proximal vascular clamp is removed and the artery controlled by finger pressure as the embolectomy is advanced into the iliac artery.

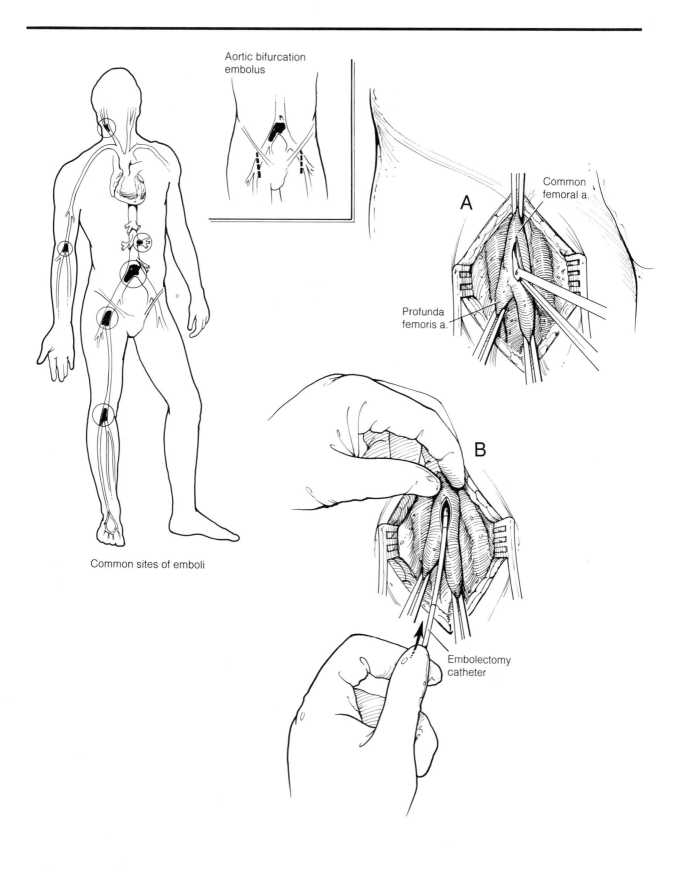

Aortic bifurcation embolus

Common sites of emboli

Common femoral a.

Profunda femoris a.

A

B

Embolectomy catheter

Fig 29-1,C. The embolectomy catheter is pushed through into the aorta above the bifurcation. The balloon is inflated above the embolic clot. The catheter is withdrawn through the iliac artery pulling the clot along with the balloon. The size of the balloon is adjusted by changing pressure on the syringe used to inflate the balloon as it passes through the arteries so that it remains occlusive with the arterial wall but not so tight that it could disrupt the intima.

D. The embolus is removed through the arteriotomy in the common femoral artery. A vessel loop passed around the femoral artery and lifted up can be used to occlude inflow, or digital pressure and the occasional reapplication of the vascular clamp proximal to the arteriotomy may be used as required for hemostasis. The embolectomy catheter is passed repeatedly until no further clot is obtained and there is vigorous blood flow from the arteriotomy.

E. The embolectomy process is repeated in the opposite groin. It is convenient to perform this procedure simultaneously from each groin. Following removal of all the embolic material, the arteriotomy is repaired by continuous suture.

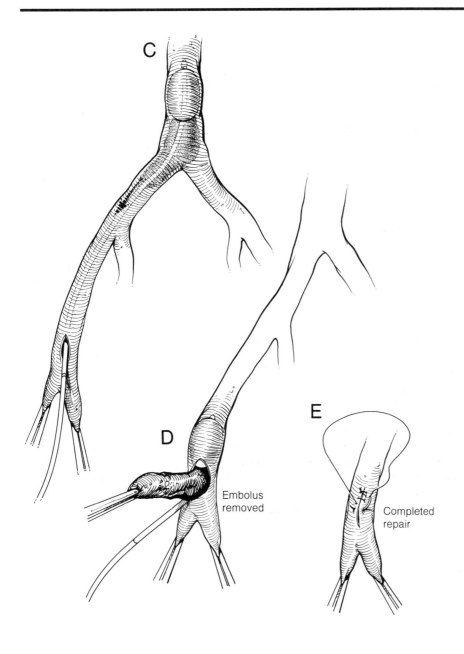

C

D

Embolus
removed

E

Completed
repair

Femoro-popliteal Arterial Embolectomy

Fig 29–2, A. Arterial emboli lodging in the bifurcation of the femoral or popliteal arteries are removed through incision in the groin over the common femoral artery. It is rarely necessary to have more distal incision of the arteries.

B. The common femoral, profunda femoris, and superficial femoral arteries are mobilized and controlled by vascular clamp. An arteriotomy is made in the common femoral artery. Embolic material is cleared from the common femoral artery. An embolectomy catheter (3F or 4F size) is introduced to the superficial femoral artery through the arteriotomy. The vascular clamp is removed from the superficial femoral artery and blood loss controlled by digital pressure on the artery. The embolectomy catheter is passed distally as far as possible. Usually it passes into the arteries in the foot.

C. The balloon is inflated and the catheter is withdrawn pulling the embolic material with it. The size of the balloon must be gradually increased as the cathether is withdrawn to keep it in contact with the arterial intima. Some resistance with the arterial intima is necessary, but the balloon should not be overinflated so that intimal disruption could occur.

D. The embolus is removed at the arteriotomy in the common femoral artery. The cathether is passed distally as many times as necessary to clear out all embolic clot. The catheter should be passed into the profunda femoris artery to assure that the deep arterial circulation is free of arterial embolus. A 5F embolectomy cathether should be passed proximally into the common femoral and iliac artery to assure inflow.

E. The arteriotomy is repaired by continuous suture. After blood flow is restored to the extremity, the integrity of the distal circulation should be evaluated by Doppler ultrasound. Palpable peripheral pulses are desirable but not always present immediately after embolectomy due to arterial spasm caused by ischemia and by the balloon catheter manipulation. It is often helpful to inject papaverine 30 mg directly into the femoral artery through a 25 gauge needle to relieve arterial spasm.

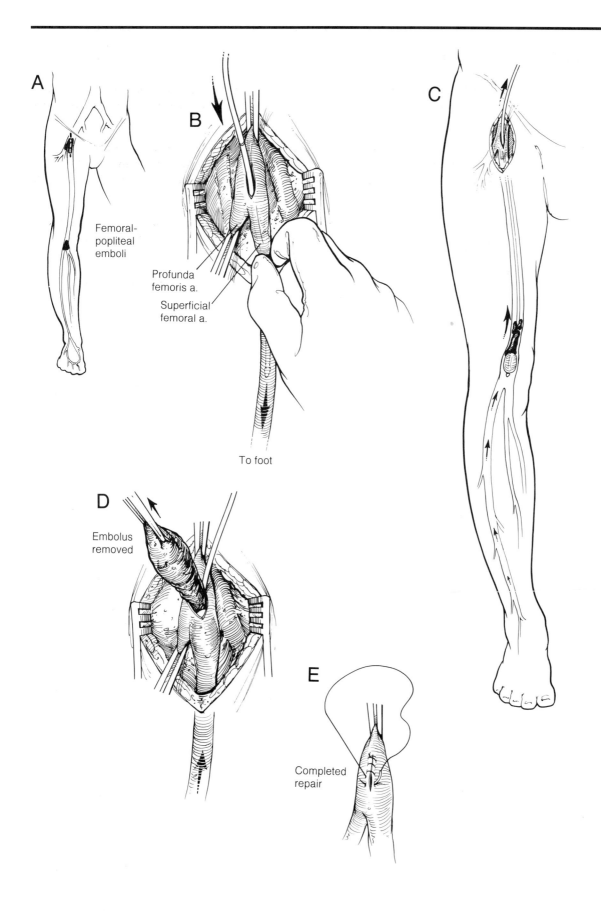

A

Femoral-
popliteal
emboli

B

Profunda
femoris a.

Superficial
femoral a.

To foot

C

D

Embolus
removed

E

Completed
repair

Brachial-radial-ulnar Arterial Embolectomy

Fig 29–3, A. Emboli to the arteries of the arm are removed through arteriotomy in the brachial artery. An "S" type incision is made in the anticubital fossa to expose the brachial artery and its bifurcation.

B. A vascular clamp is applied to the brachial artery proximally. Distally, it is controlled above the bifurcation with a Silastic vessel loop. An arteriotomy is made and the embolectomy catheter introduced. The catheter is passed as far distally as possible to the arteries of the hand.

C. The balloon is inflated and the catheter withdrawn. The embolus is removed from the arteriotomy as the balloon delivers it to that point. The catheter is passed into the arterial system until all clot is removed as indicated by one or two clear passes.

D. The arteriotomy is repaired by continuous suture. The distal circulation is evaluated by Doppler ultrasound after blood flow is restored.

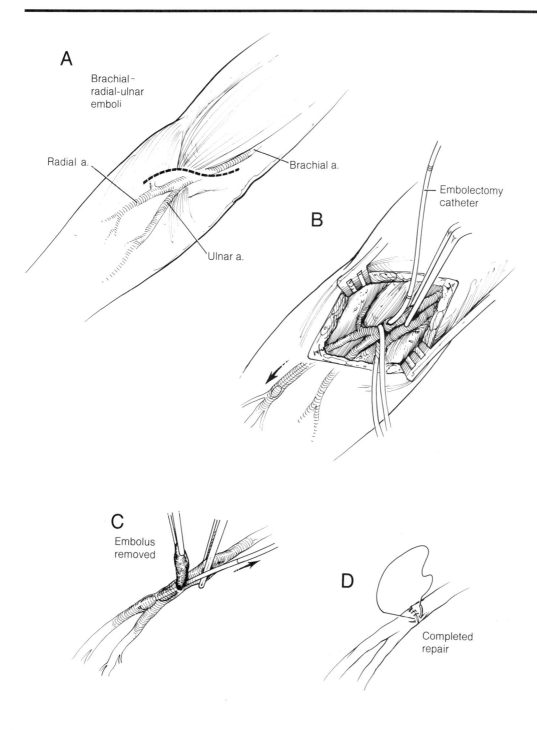

A

Brachial-
radial-ulnar
emboli

Radial a.

Brachial a.

Ulnar a.

B

Embolectomy
catheter

C

Embolus
removed

D

Completed
repair

30

Fasciotomy

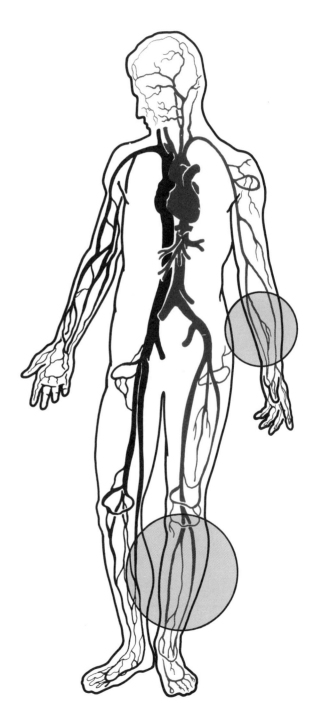

Fig 30–1. Reperfusion of the ischemic extremity often results in swelling of the tissues temporarily injured by lack of blood flow. The muscles of the extremities are enveloped by fascia that may restrict swelling. Extreme swelling of muscles of the extremities may cause pressure within the fascial compartments to rise sufficiently to exceed arterial input and again render the muscles in the compartment ischemic. Excessively high pressure may compress nerves and their blood supply resulting in permanent neural damage.

A. Cross-sectional anatomy of the leg shows the division of the muscles by fascia and the interosseous membrane into four compartments: (1) the anterior compartment containing the tibialis and extensor digitorum longus; (2) the lateral compartment containing the peroneus longus; (3) the deep posterior compartment containing the tibialis posterior, popliteus, and flexor digitorum longus; and (4) the posterior compartment containing the gastrocnemius and soleus muscles. The anterior and lateral compartments are often considered together because they are separated from the rest by the interosseous membrane. The anterior tibial artery and the deep peroneal nerve lie on the interosseous membrane and are subject to compression by the muscles of the anterior and lateral compartment. The deep posterior and posterior compartments are behind the interosseous membrane and may compress the posterior tibial artery and the tibial nerve.

B. Complete decompression of the muscle compartments of the leg is possible by removal of a segment of the fibula. This maneuver releases the interosseous membrane along with the compartment muscle-fascia attachments, allowing the muscle compartments to expand into the wound laterally.

C. A longitudinal incision is made over the fibula on the lateral aspect of the leg, taking care to avoid the peroneal nerve as it courses around the head of the fibula. Dissection is taken onto the fibula. The periostium is elevated and about one-third of the fibula is excised. No functional loss occurs with fibulectomy.

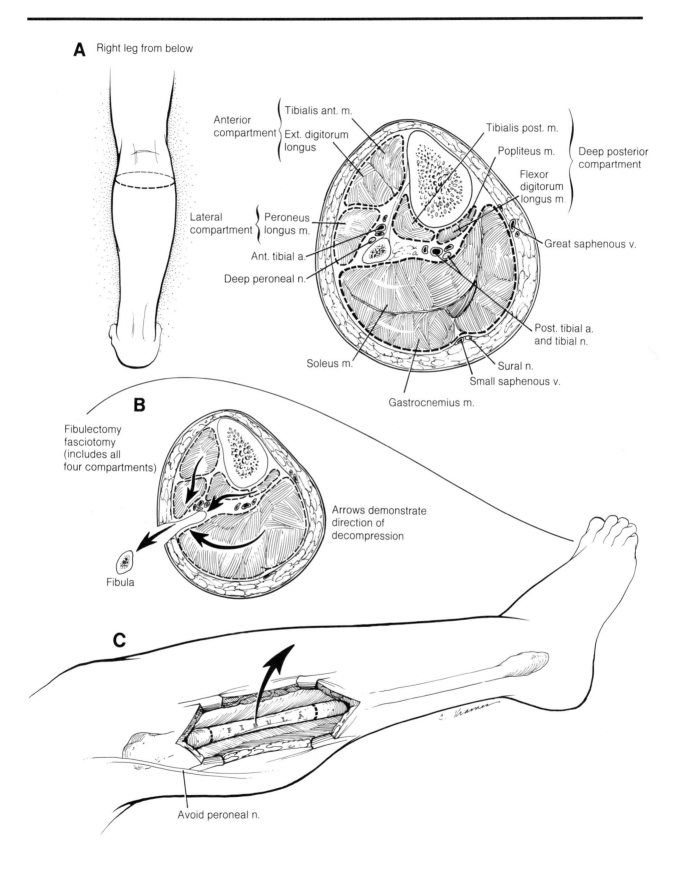

A Right leg from below

Anterior compartment { Tibialis ant. m.
Ext. digitorum longus

Lateral compartment { Peroneus longus m.

Ant. tibial a.

Deep peroneal n.

Tibialis post. m.
Popliteus m.
Flexor digitorum longus m.

Deep posterior compartment

Great saphenous v.

Post. tibial a. and tibial n.

Soleus m.

Sural n.
Small saphenous v.

Gastrocnemius m.

B

Fibulectomy fasciotomy (includes all four compartments)

Arrows demonstrate direction of decompression

Fibula

C

Avoid peroneal n.

Fibula

Limited Fasciotomy

Anterior Compartment Fasciotomy

Fig 30–2, A. Decompression of the anterior compartment independent of the rest of the compartments is accomplished through a moderate length skin incision over the anterior compartment alongside the tibia.

B. This incision will come down on the fascia that envelopes the tibialis anterior and the extensor digitorum longus muscles.

C. The skin incision allows the muscle-fascia to bulge into the wound. A longer skin incision may be made if the skin seems restrictive.

D. The fascial sheath is opened as far up and down the leg as possible by inserting the blades of partially opened scissors beneath the fascial edge and pushing ahead to incise the fascia and undermine the skin.

Limited Fasciotomy:

Anterior
Compartment
Fasciotomy

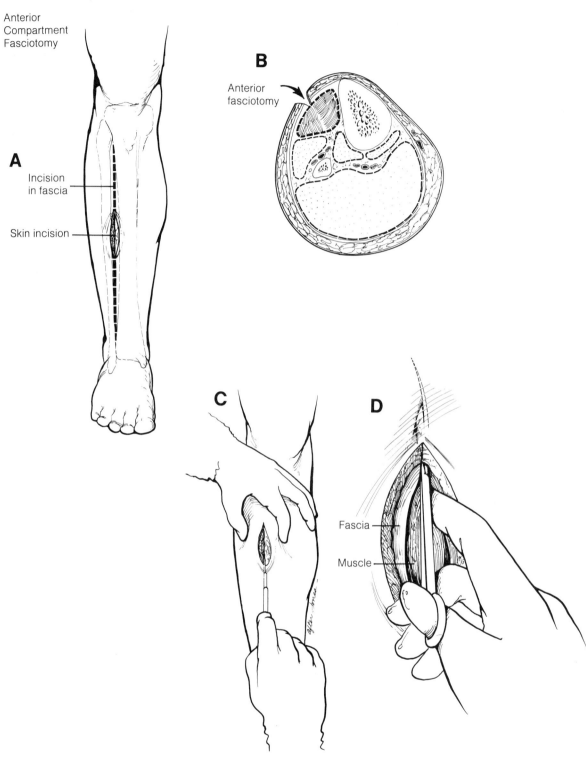

A

Incision
in fascia

Skin incision

B

Anterior
fasciotomy

C

D

Fascia

Muscle

Lateral Compartment Fasciotomy

Fig 30–3, A. An incision on the lateral aspect of the leg just anterior to the fibula will come down on the fascial sheath of the lateral compartment containing the peroneus longus muscle.

B. The fascial sheath is incised and scissors advanced the length of the compartment beneath the skin.

Posterior Compartment Fasciotomy

A. An incision on the posterior aspect of the leg will encounter the enveloping fascia of the posterior compartment.

B. The fascial sheath is incised and scissors pushed the length of the calf to completely open up the fascia of the posterior compartment.

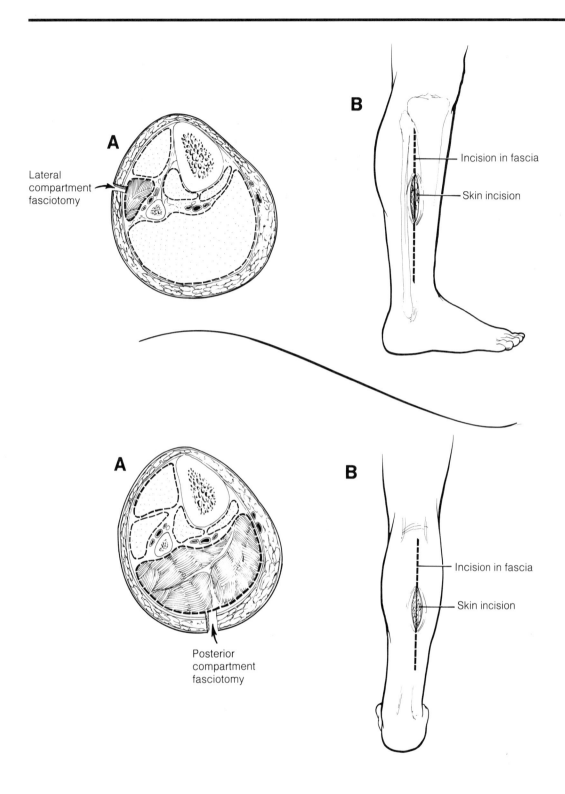

A

Lateral
compartment
fasciotomy

B

Incision in fascia

Skin incision

A

Posterior
compartment
fasciotomy

B

Incision in fascia

Skin incision

Forearm Fasciotomy

Fig 30–4.   Relief of compartment swelling in the forearm is accomplished by incision of the fascia on the volar and dorsal surfaces of the arm.

A.   Anterior fasciotomy is done through a longitudinal skin incision near the middle of the volar surface of the forearm. Scissors are advanced through the fascial sheath up and down the arm to widely open the fascia and undermine the skin.

B.   Posterior fasciotomy is done through a longitudinal skin incision on the dorsal surface of the forearm. The fascia is opened widely by pushing scissors under the skin the length of the forearm.

C.   Cross-section of the forearm shows how anterior and posterior incision of the fascial compartments will decompress swelling in the forearm.

Forearm Fasciotomy

A   Anterior

B   Posterior

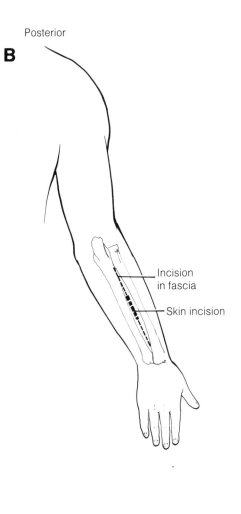

Incision
in fascia

Skin incision

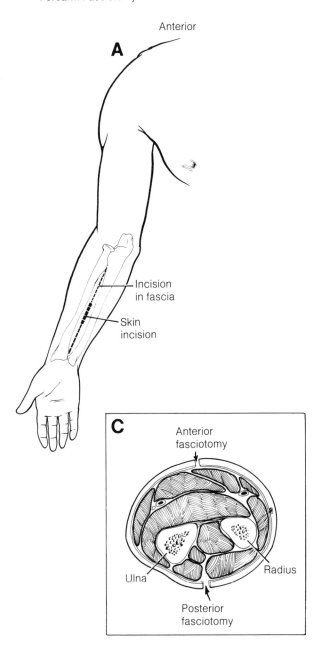

Incision
in fascia

Skin
incision

C   Anterior
     fasciotomy

Ulna

Radius

Posterior
fasciotomy

Amputation

31

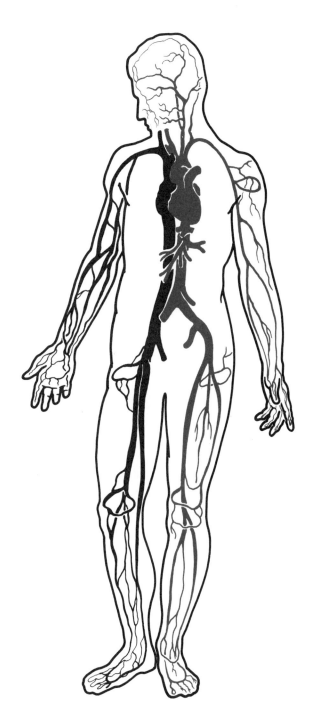

Above-knee Amputation

Fig 31–1. Amputation is a procedure that vascular surgeons do not like to perform because it represents either failure of reconstructive vascular operation or an anatomic situation not amenable to revascularization procedures. Nevertheless, these procedures often represent significant rehabilitative measures when a limb is dead and may be a great relief to patients suffering from pain.

A. Above-knee amputation is performed through a circumferential incision above the knee preserving as much skin length as is feasible.

B. The deep tissue incision progresses back to bone approximately 5 cm above the skin incision.

C. The deep fascia is incised 2 cm proximal to the skin incision in circumferential fashion.

D. The muscle anterior to the femur is divided anterior and lateral to the bone progressing to a point about 5 cm above the skin incision. The periosteum is elevated from the femur. A Gigli saw is passed around the femur. The bone is divided.

E. With the bone separated, the popliteal neurovascular bundle may be identified. The popliteal artery and veins are divided.

F. The sciatic nerve is ligated proximally and divided to prevent bleeding from the perineural blood supply and the formation of neuroma.

G. The hamstring muscle group is divided posteriorly with a large amputation knife.

H. Cross-sectional anatomy of the thigh calls attention to the location of the popliteal artery and veins and the sciatic nerve posterior to the femur.

I. The deep fascia is approximated transversely with interrupted stitches of absorbable suture material.

J. Meticulous skin closure with multiple small interrupted stitches is then performed. Verticle mattress stitches are avoided because of the tendency of this technique to interrupt blood supply to the skin edge.

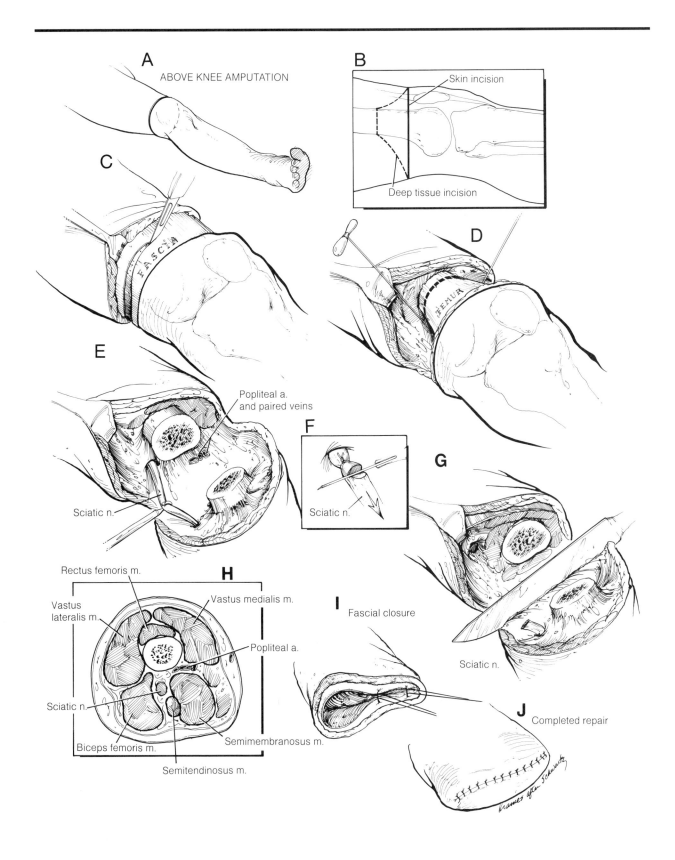

A ABOVE KNEE AMPUTATION

B
Skin incision
Deep tissue incision

C FASCIA

D FEMUR

E
Popliteal a. and paired veins
Sciatic n.

F
Sciatic n.

G
Sciatic n.

H
Rectus femoris m.
Vastus lateralis m.
Vastus medialis m.
Popliteal a.
Sciatic n.
Biceps femoris m.
Semimembranosus m.
Semitendinosus m.

I Fascial closure

J Completed repair

Below-knee Amputation

Fig 31–2, A. Amputation of the leg below the knee is performed through a transverse anterior skin incision with a long posterior flap that has better blood supply. The incision should be carefully planned so that the posterior skin flap is long enough to cover the amputation site without tension. The point of division of the tibia should be about two finger-breadths below the tubercle. The anterior skin flap should be an additional two finger-breadths below that point.

B. Dissection is taken deep to the fascia so that a flap of skin, subcutaneous tissue, and fascia is raised. The dissection is to the level of the tibia anteriorly.

C. The muscle of the anterior compartment group is divided. The anterior tibial artery and vein are usually encountered and must be ligated. The tibia and fibula are freed of muscle attachments by elevation of the periosteum from the bone circumferentially. A Gigli saw is used to divide the fibula. The fibula is divided approximately 2 cm proximal to the level selected for division of the tibia.

D. The tibia is divided and the anterior aspect cut back as a bevel to eliminate sharpness of the bone. The posterior muscle groups are divided well distal to the point of bone division by amputation knife. Sufficient length is maintained on the posterior muscle to allow coverage of the bone. If the flap is too thick and bulky, the soleum muscle may be excised leaving the gastrocnemius muscle.

E. Hemostasis is obtained in the cut end of the muscle. The fascia is closed with interrupted stitches of absorbable suture.

F. The skin closure is by small interrupted stitches of fine monofilament suture material (wire, nylon, or polypropylene). The suture line is anterior with a pad of muscle and skin from the posterior flap covering the bone ends.

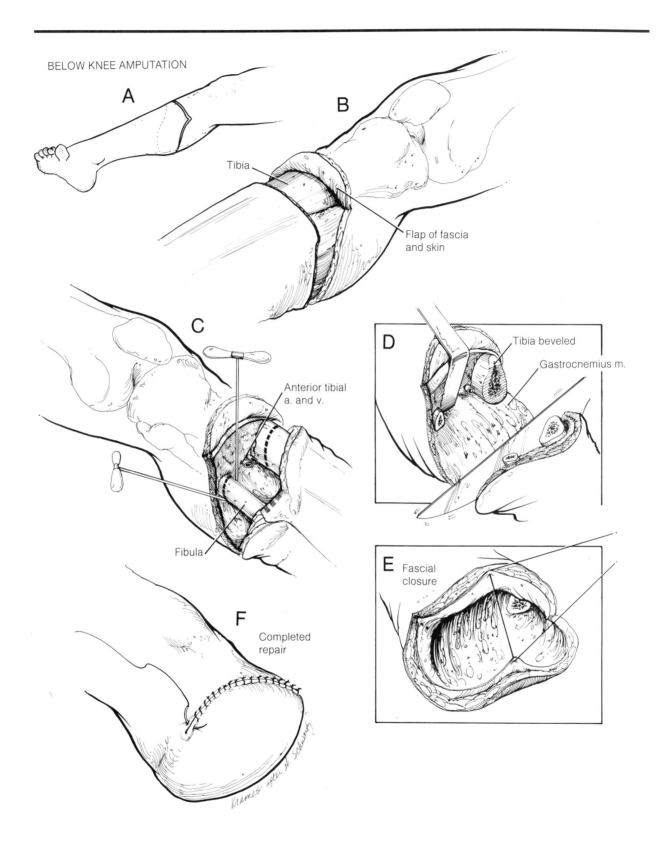

A

B

Tibia

Flap of fascia
and skin

C

Anterior tibial
a. and v.

Fibula

D

Tibia beveled

Gastrocnemius m.

E Fascial
closure

F

Completed
repair

Transmetatarsal Amputation of Toes

Fig 31–3, A. The skin incision on the dorsal surface of the foot is just proximal to the metatarsal heads.

B. On the plantar surface, the incision is near the base of the toes, preserving as much of the plantar weight-bearing surface as possible.

C. The incision is continued down to the bone.

D. Plantar flexion of the toes and downward traction aids the incision and dissection which divides the extensor tendons of the toes.

E. A plantar flap of tendon, subcutaneous fat, and deep fascia is developed along with the skin back proximal to the metatarsal heads.

F. Periosteum is elevated from the metatarsal bones. A Gigli saw is used to divide the metatarsals proximal to the heads.

G. The completed amputation should maintain a sufficient plantar flap to allow closure of the foot anterior to the bones.

H. The deep fascia is reapproximated with interrupted stitches of absorbable suture.

I. Skin closure is by meticulous simple interrupted stitches of fine monofilament suture material.

TRANSMETATARSAL AMPUTATION OF TOES

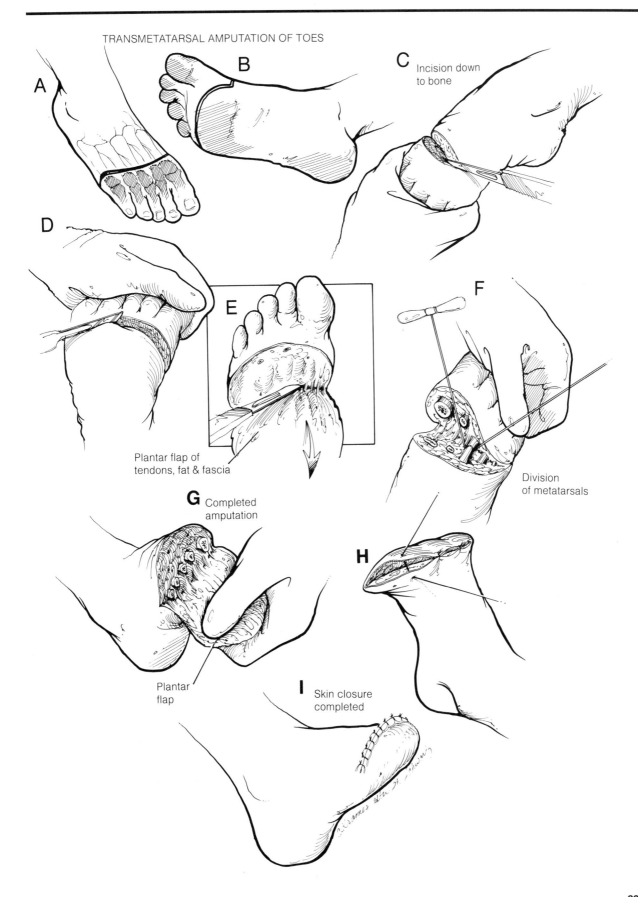

A

B

C Incision down to bone

D

E

Plantar flap of tendons, fat & fascia

F

Division of metatarsals

G Completed amputation

Plantar flap

H

I Skin closure completed

Transmetatarsal Amputation of Toes One or Five

Fig 31–4, A. The first or fifth toe may be removed by transmetatarsal amputation. A racket-shaped incision is started on the dorsal surface of the foot just proximal to the first metatarsal head. The incision crosses the metatarsal and is taken into the groove between the first and second toes.

B. On the plantar surface, the incision is at the base of the toe so as to preserve as much of the plantar weight-bearing surface as possible.

C. Medially, the incisions approximate each other and join just above the metatarsal head.

D. The metatarsal bone is divided proximal to the head. The soft tissue is divided while maintaining as much skin and fascia as possible on the plantar surface to complete the amputation of the toe. The skin is reapproximated anteriorly with multiple small interrupted stitches of fine monofilament suture material.

Transphalangeal Amputation of Second, Third, or Fourth Toes

A. Necrosis of the second, third, or fourth toes is usually treated by simply removing the phalanx. A skin incision is made around the base of the toe preserving as much of the skin on each lateral aspect as possible. The bone is divided at the base of the proximal phalanx.

B. The skin edges are approximated vertically.

TRANSMETATARSAL AMPUTATION (of 1st and 5th toes)

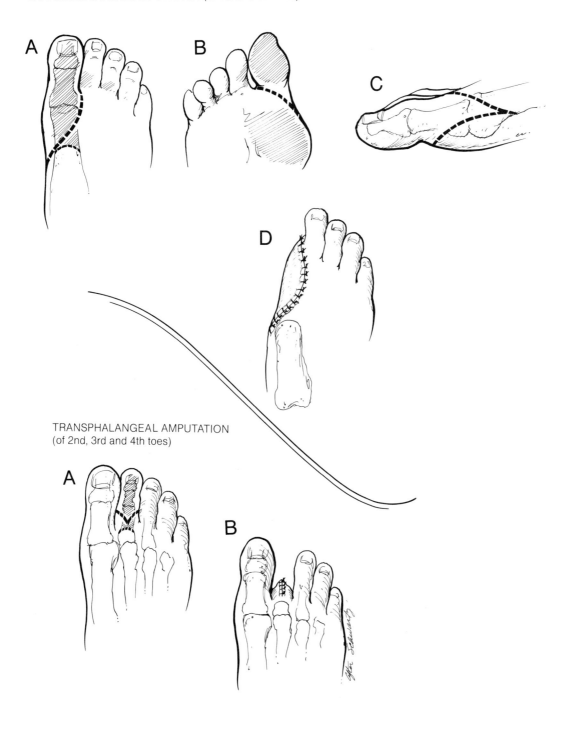

TRANSPHALANGEAL AMPUTATION
(of 2nd, 3rd and 4th toes)

Sympathectomy

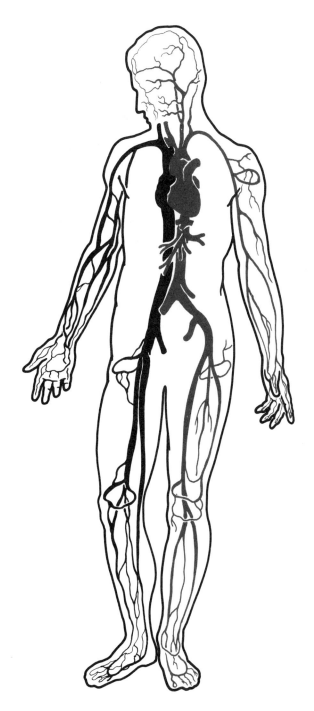

32

Lumbar Sympathectomy

Fig 32–1. Excision of the lumbar sympathetic neural chain is performed through a flank incision. The incision is placed lateral to the rectus sheath about the level of the umbilicus extending laterally in a transverse fashion to about the posterior axillary line. The patient may be positioned with a roll under the hip to bring the flank into a more anterior position.

A. A muscle-splitting incision is employed. The external oblique muscle is opened parallel to the fascial fibers from the edge of the rectus sheath into the flank. The muscle fibers of the internal oblique and transversus abdominus muscles are separated to expose the preperitoneal space.

B. The peritoneum is swept away from the muscles of the posterior abdominal wall and back. An effort is made to keep the peritoneum intact so that the abdominal contents are contained. The dissection proceeds across the psoas muscle to the inferior vena cava. The ureter and gonadal vessels are taken anteriorly with the peritoneum and its contents. The vertebral bodies are identified. Lumbar arteries and veins are identified and preserved as they course laterally and posteriorly over the spine. The genitofemoral nerve located on the psoas muscle is identified, preserved, and not confused with the sympathetic chain. The lumbar sympathetic neural chain is identified alongside the spine.

C. The lumbar sympathetic chain is excised. The sacral promontory is a useful landmark as L4 sympathetic ganglion lies just above the promontory and L3 is above that. Both these ganglia should be removed along with L5 ganglion. If technically feasible, L2 ganglion is included in the resection, but L1 ganglion is not removed to prevent problems with ejaculation in men. Hemoclips are placed across the neural chain at the limits of excision.

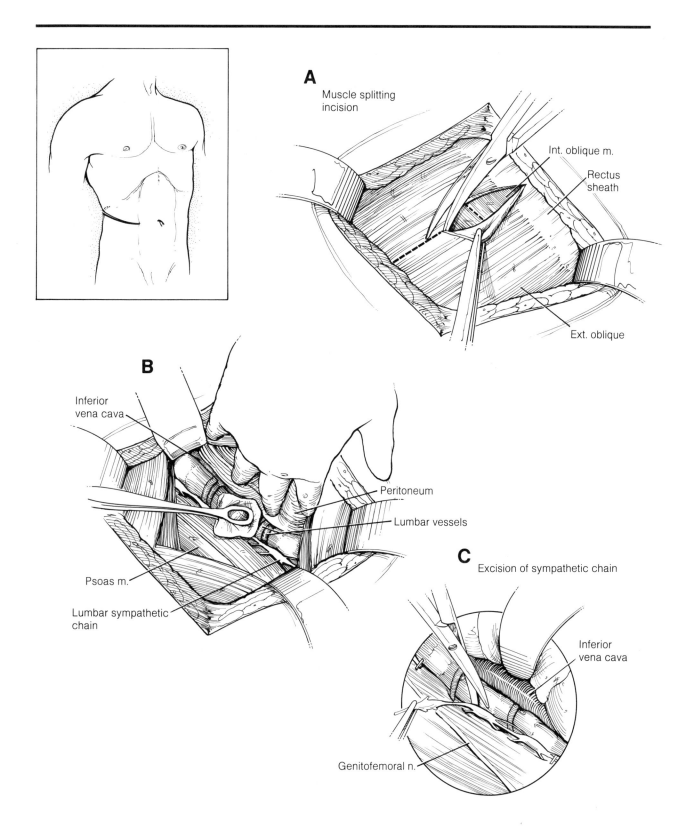

A

Muscle splitting incision

Int. oblique m.

Rectus sheath

Ext. oblique

B

Inferior vena cava

Peritoneum

Lumbar vessels

Psoas m.

Lumbar sympathetic chain

C

Excision of sympathetic chain

Inferior vena cava

Genitofemoral n.

Thoracic Sympathectomy

Fig 32–2. Excision of the thoracic sympathetic neural chain is performed through an axillary incision. A transverse incision is made in the axilla at the lower margin of the hairline. The incision extends from the posterior border of the pectoralis major to the anterior border of the latissimus dorsi. A longer incision is of no advantage because the muscles limit the exposure. The arm is draped into the operating field so that an assistant can maintain reasonably comfortable retraction to relax the axillary fossa.

A. The axillary fat pad is retracted toward the arm so that the dissection may proceed directly to the chest wall. The intercostobrachialis nerve is identified and protected from injury to avoid numbness of the medial aspect of the upper arm. The second rib is identified and an incision made in the periosteum with electrocautery.

B. The periosteum is elevated from the inferior margin of the second rib. The pleural space is opened through the bed of the nonresected rib.

C. A thoracotomy retractor is used to separate the ribs. The lung is retracted inferiorly to expose the apex of the pleural space. The spine is identified. The parietal pleura is opened over the lateral aspect of the upper thoracic spine. The thoracic sympathetic chain is identified and its ganglia exposed. The stellate ganglion lies opposite the first thoracic vertebra over the head of the first rib. It should be identified and dissected out completely to determine its complete length. Only the lower one-third or half of the stellate ganglion is removed.

D. The sympathetic chain is removed including three to five ganglia. A hemoclip is used to mark the extent of the excision.

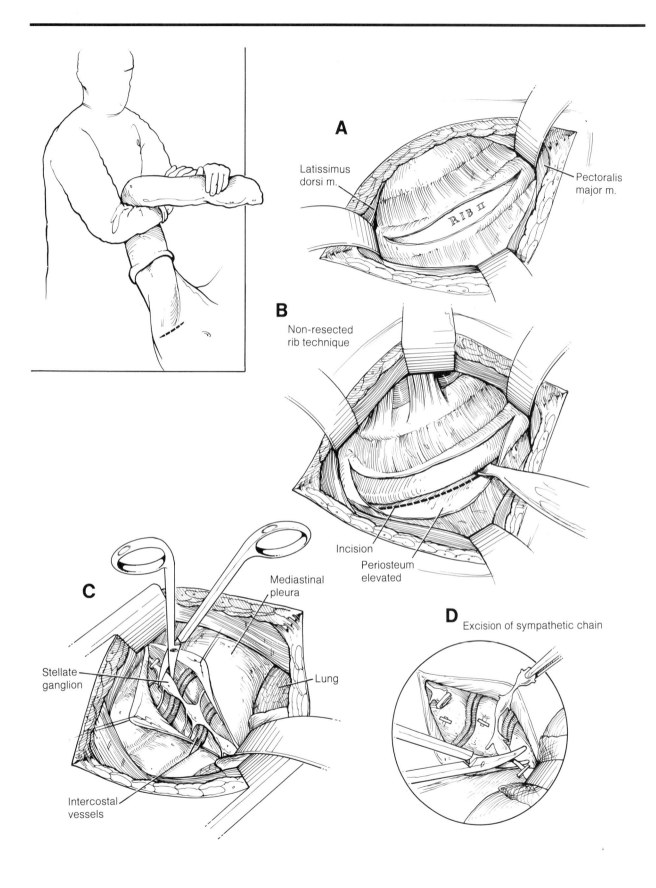

A

Latissimus dorsi m.

Pectoralis major m.

RIB II

B

Non-resected rib technique

Incision

Periosteum elevated

C

Stellate ganglion

Intercostal vessels

Mediastinal pleura

Lung

D Excision of sympathetic chain

Thoracic Outlet
Compression Syndrome

33

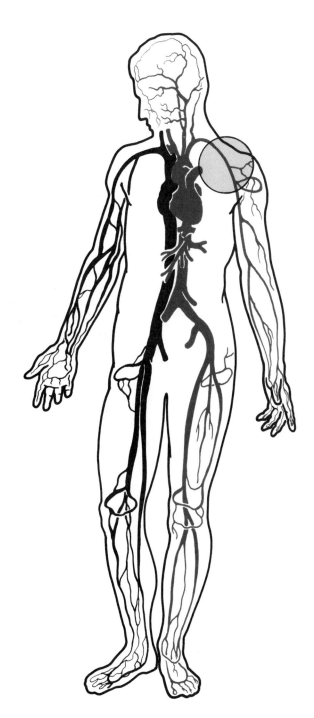

First Rib Resection

Fig 33–1. Resection of the first rib for thoracic outlet compression syndrome is a somewhat controversial though widely practiced operation. The patient with chronic pain in the arm and numbness in the ulnar nerve distribution is most likely to have relief of symptoms with this operation.

A transaxillary approach is used. Anterior, posterior, and supraclavicular approaches have been described, but the transaxillary one seems to combine the least operative disability with adequate exposure. The patient is placed in the lateral thoracotomy position on the operating table, and the chest, axilla, and arm on the affected side are prepared. The arm is draped into the operating field so that an assistant may grasp the arm with the elbow bent and retract it anteriorly. Interlocking the arms of the patient and the assistant at the elbow makes the assistant's job easier. A skin line transverse incision is made in the axilla at the lower border of the axillary hair line. The excision extends from the posterior border of the pectoralis major muscle to the anterior border of the latissimus dorsi muscle. A longer incision does not enhance the exposure to any appreciable degree and reduces the cosmetic value once beyond the muscle borders described.

A. The neurovascular bundle to the arm is compressed in the thoracic outlet syndrome between the first rib, clavicle, and the scalene muscles. Resection of the first rib not only removes the bony rib and allows the neurovascular bundle to settle down to the second rib but also releases the muscle attachments of the scalenus anticus and medius.

B. The skin and subcutaneous tissues are divided and retracted. The axillary fat pad should not be entered; its lymphatics and fat are retracted superiorly. The dissection is taken to the chest wall and the loose areolar tissue over the ribs swept away. In the course of the dissection, the intercostobrachialis nerve is identified coming out of the second interspace and taking a course through the axilla out onto the medial aspect of the arm. This nerve should be carefully preserved to avoid numbness of the upper inner aspect of the arm and axilla. This nerve is also a good guide to the second rib and thus helps identify with surety the first rib to be removed. The scalene muscles partly obscure the neurovascular bundle at this point, but the pulsations of the axillary artery are easily palpable.

C. The periosteum of the first rib is incised with the electrocautery. The scalene muscles are cut away from the first rib with the electrocautery or with the dissection of the periosteum.

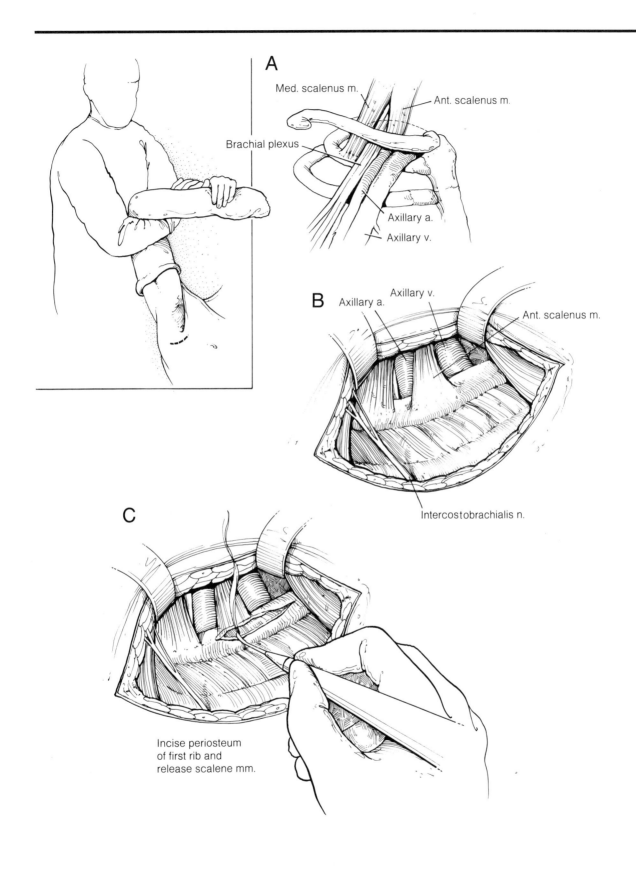

A

Med. scalenus m.

Ant. scalenus m.

Brachial plexus

Axillary a.

Axillary v.

B

Axillary a.

Axillary v.

Ant. scalenus m.

Intercostobrachialis n.

C

Incise periosteum
of first rib and
release scalene mm.

Fig 33–1, D. A periosteal elevator is used to remove the periosteum completely from the first rib. It is important to stay in the subperiosteal plane to avoid penetration of the pleural space. The periosteal resection should be performed deliberately and patiently to obtain as much exposure to the length of the first rib as possible.

E. The first rib is divided anteriorly as close as possible to the manubrium of the sternum using rib shears.

F. The rib is retracted appropriately by a Kocher clamp on the anterior cut edge to allow placement of first rib shears as posterior as possible on the rib. The rib is divided posteriorly as near to the spine as possible. Care is taken to retract the brachial plexus as needed using a nerve hook when closing the rib shears for the posterior rib division. Only a small spur of the posterior attachment of the rib should remain when it is divided. Occasionally, box-cut rib shears are required to trim back the remaining rib to obtain maximum rib removal.

The neurovascular bundle to the arm is completely decompressed as it is allowed to drop down to the second rib and the scalene muscles retract away from it.

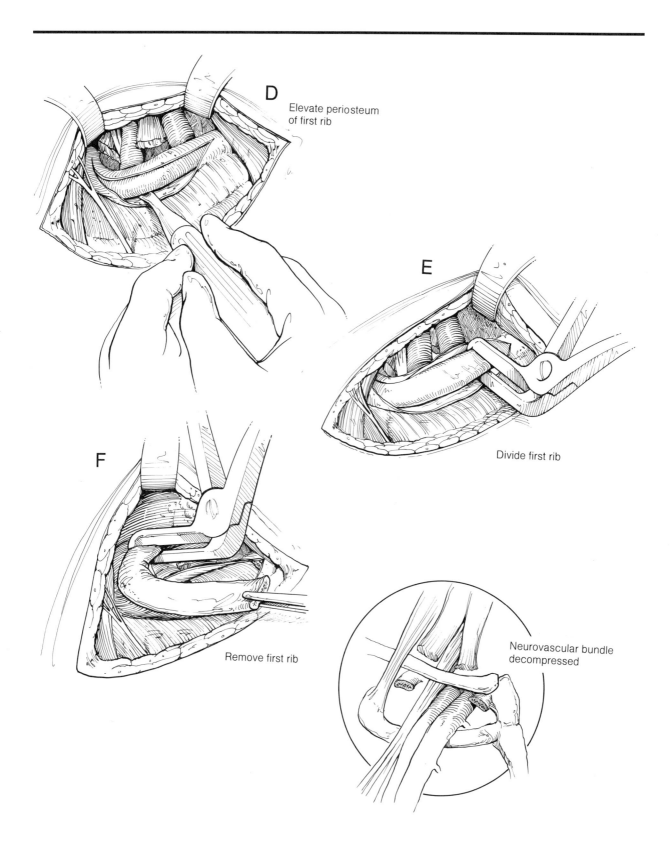

D

Elevate periosteum
of first rib

E

Divide first rib

F

Remove first rib

Neurovascular bundle
decompressed

Bypass of Superior Vena Cava

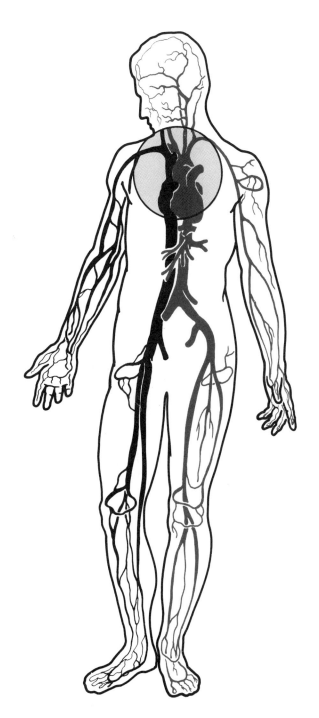

Fig 34–1, A. A midsternal incision is made. The incision may be extended into the neck with division of the strap muscles on either side to obtain access to the internal jugular vein if necessary. Chest wall collateral circulation is controlled by electrocautery. An autotransfusion device-cell saver is helpful in reducing blood replacement requirements. Once it has been determined that bypass operation is feasible, an incision is made in the leg over the saphenous vein.

B. A biopsy of the obstructing process in the mediastinum is taken. The upper portion of the pericardium is opened in the midline to expose the right atrial appendage. The thymic remnant is removed and the innominate vein is completely mobilized. When the internal jugular veins are used as the input site, the strap muscles on that side should be removed to open up the thoracic inlet as much as possible.

Construction of Composite Spiral Saphenous Vein Graft

C. The spiral vein graft should be precisely the same diameter as the vein to which it is to be anastomosed and exactly long enough to span between the vein and the right atrial appendage. There is no advantage to extra length which may cause the graft to kink. As a practical matter, the saphenous vein excised from groin to knee will be just about right for a graft 12 mm in diameter which will span between the innominate vein and right atrial appendage. The saphenous vein is distended with heparinized saline solution and all side branches are ligated. The vein is opened longitudinally through its entire length. An argyle thoracostomy catheter that is exactly the same size as the vein to which the graft will be anastomosed is chosen to form the stent on which the composite graft will be constructed. The opened saphenous vein is then wrapped around the stent catheter in spiral fashion with the intimal surface against the stent and maintaining orientation of the direction of the valves. The edges of the saphenous vein are joined by continuous suture of 7/0 polypropylene, forming a spiral anastomosis the length of the graft.

D. Heparin, 100–200 units kg, is administered intravenously to the patient. The innominate vein is ligated as close to the superior vena cava as possible. A soft jaw vascular clamp (Fogarty) is applied at the jugular-subclavian vein confluence and the innominate vein divided so that as much length as possible is preserved. The end of the composite graft is pushed slightly off the end of the stent. An end-to-end anastomosis of the graft to the innominate vein is constructed with continuous stitches of 7/0 polypropylene suture. When the anastomosis is complete, the stent is removed.

E. The entire right atrial appendage is excluded by vascular clamp, the tip of the appendage excised, and all trabeculae within the appendage are removed.

F. The end of the vein graft is anastomosed to the right atrial appendage with 5/0 polypropylene suture.

G. The completed graft lies anterior to the aorta. The pericardium is left open; wound closure is routine.

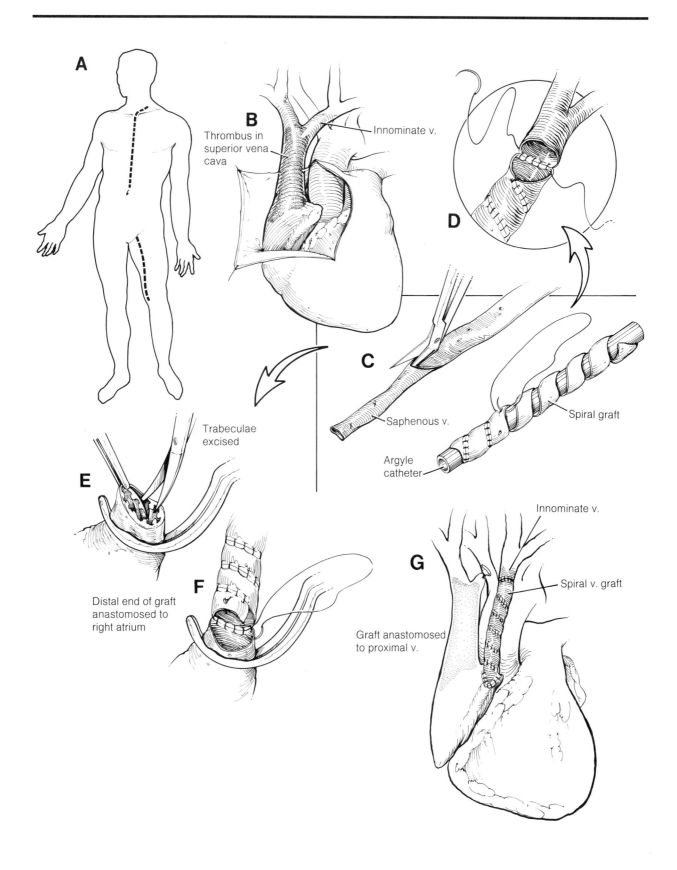

A

B
Thrombus in superior vena cava

Innominate v.

D

C

Saphenous v.

Argyle catheter

Spiral graft

E
Trabeculae excised

Distal end of graft anastomosed to right atrium

F

G
Innominate v.

Spiral v. graft

Graft anastomosed to proximal v.

Venous Insufficiency

35

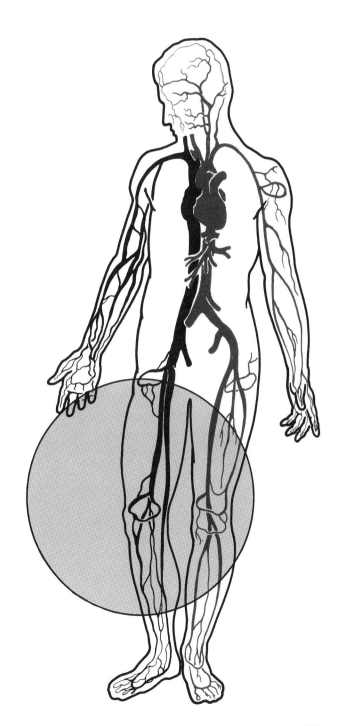

Varicose Vein Ligation/Stripping

Fig 35–1. Ectasia and tortuosity of superficial veins of the leg resulting in venous valve incompetence and "varicose" veins is a common problem encountered in vascular surgery. These enlarged veins are not only unsightly and a bad cosmetic problem, but the venous stasis changes associated with them may result in difficult skin problems with pigmentation changes, ulceration, and bleeding from the exposed varicosities. The greater saphenous vein system on the anterior and medial surface of the leg are most commonly affected, but the short or lesser saphenous system on the posterior and lateral surface of the leg may be involved below the knee where this vein joins the popliteal vein of the deep venous system. This junction point is at the upper end of the popliteal fossa above the skin crease of the knee.

Greater Saphenous Strapping

A. Stripping of the greater saphenous vein should be performed only if there are varicose changes of this vein. In some cases, the main greater saphenous channel is normal and it is really the superficial branches of the vein which are abnormal. Incisions are made in the groin just below the inguinal ligament over the femoral vein and at the ankle just anterior to the medial malleolus. Transverse skin incisions are preferred which are only as long as necessary to achieve adequate exposure.

B. The saphenous vein is freed from surrounding alveolar tissue. The saphenous nerve is closely associated with the vein and should be separated from it.

C. The vein is ligated distally and the catheter of the stripper device passed proximally through the lumen of the saphenous vein. Hopefully, the stripper will find its way to the groin incision inside the saphenous vein. In some cases the vein is so tortuous that this is not possible. Another incision must then be made over the vein at the point where the stripper can no longer be advanced.

D. The obturator of the stripper device is attached to the catheter and the vein tightly secured to the stripper by ligature.

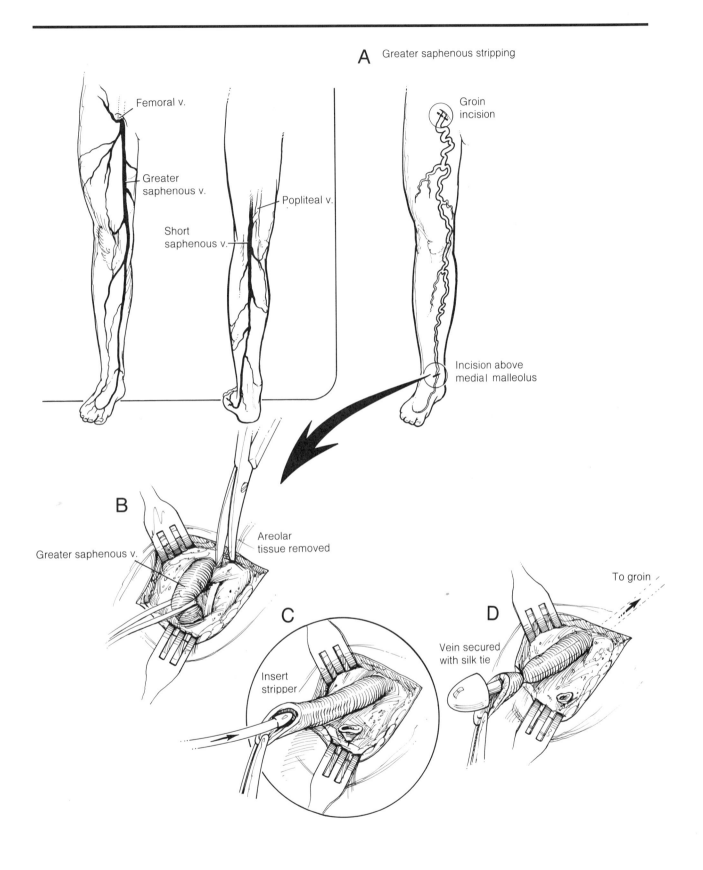

A Greater saphenous stripping

Femoral v.

Greater
saphenous v.

Short
saphenous v.

Popliteal v.

Groin
incision

Incision above
medial malleolus

B

Greater saphenous v.

Areolar
tissue removed

C

Insert
stripper

D

To groin

Vein secured
with silk tie

Fig 35–1, E. The saphenous vein and its branches are dissected in the groin. The femoral vein junction must be accurately identified and all the proximal side branches controlled, ligated, and divided.

F. The saphenous vein is ligated and divided close to the femoral vein. The stripper catheter is retrieved from the lumen of the vein. The leg is elevated. Strong traction is applied to the stripper so that it is gradually withdrawn through the leg removing the saphenous vein with it. Pressure is applied to the vein tract sequentially as the stripper is advanced through the leg. Folded laparotomy pads are tightly pressed to the skin to control hemorrhage into the tissues. The pressure and leg elevation is continued for about five minutes or until adequate hemostasis is assured. The skin incisions are closed by subcutaneous and subcuticular stitches using absorbable suture. Strip tape is applied to obtain optimal skin approximation. The leg is washed, tincture of Benzoin applied, and small dressings applied to the skin incisions. The leg is dressed by wrapping from toes to groin with elastic adhesive. This dressing is left in place for 7–10 days. The leg is kept elevated for 24–48 hours.

Short Saphenous Stripping

A. Stripping of the short saphenous venous system is done in a manner similar to that of the great saphenous system. If only the short system is to be done, it is most easily accomplished with the patient in the prone position. Skin incisions are made in the popliteal fossa above the skinfold of the knee and posterior to the lateral malleolus at the knee.

B. The short saphenous vein is freed up at the ankle, ligated distally, divided, and the stripper catheter passed proximally to the popliteal fossa through the lumen of the vein.

C. The dissection of the short saphenous vein in the popliteal fossa should be accurate to identify the junction point of the saphenous and the popliteal vein. The superficial system may course proximally further than this junction point. The junction point must be carefully identified so that all of the saphenous vein may be removed in order to avoid leaving a short segment of varicosity behind the knee.

D. The saphenous vein is ligated flush with the popliteal vein, divided, and the stripper retrieved from the lumen. The short saphenous vein is then removed by stripping from the leg. Skin compression, closure, and dressings are managed as for greater saphenous stripping.

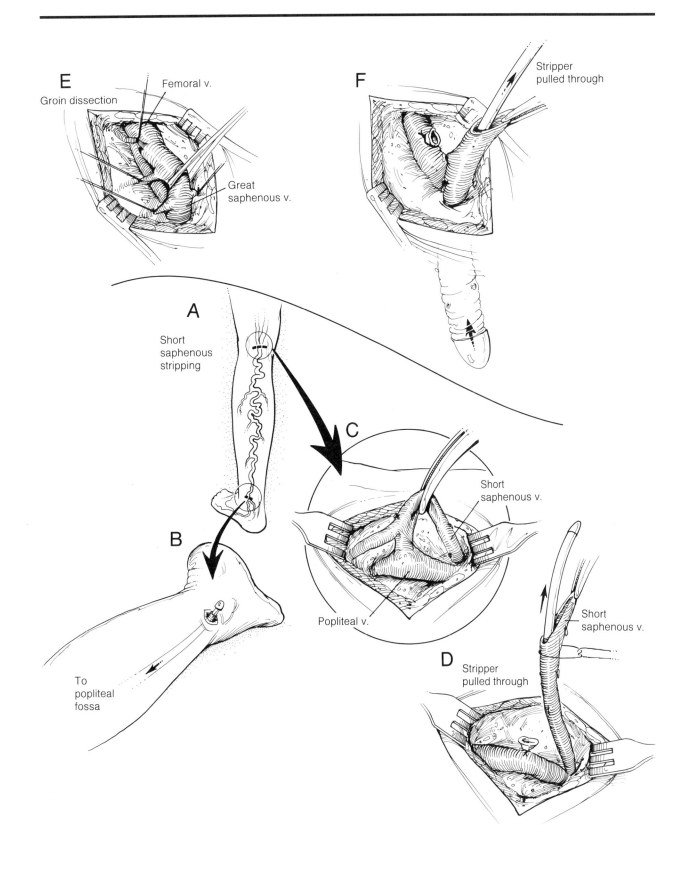

E

Groin dissection

Femoral v.

Great
saphenous v.

F

Stripper
pulled through

A

Short
saphenous
stripping

B

To
popliteal
fossa

C

Short
saphenous v.

Popliteal v.

D

Stripper
pulled through

Short
saphenous v.

Stripping of Tributary Veins

Fig 35–2, A.   Stripping of tributary veins is performed through separate incisions over the nests of varicose veins adjacent to the greater or lesser saphenous veins. In some cases, this tributary stripping process is the definitive operation and the saphenous vein is left intact when it is normal. The location of the varicose veins and the incisions to be made are done with the patient standing prior to the operation. The actual site of incision is marked by lightly scratching the skin with a 25-gauge needle. Transverse skin incisions are preferred. As many incisions as necessary to remove all of the varicosities are made.

B.   A subcutaneous dissection of the vein to be removed is made, exposing as much of the vein as can be conveniently mobilized through the incision.

C.   A curved hemostat is used to further dissect the vein in the unexposed subcutaneous tissue.

D.   The varicose vein is grasped as far into the subcutaneous tissue as possible and extracted. Hemostasis is achieved by local pressure with the leg elevated. The incisions are closed using absorbable suture in the subcutaneous and subcuticular layers. The legs are dressed as described for greater saphenous vein stripping.

Injection Therapy

Venous spiders are removed by injection therapy. These vascular structures are located in the dermis and are impossible to excise. Injection of sclerosing solution into these veins provides a treatment for an unsightly cosmetic problem. In some patients, these spiders may cover large portions of the skin of the thigh and leg. Leg make-up cremes may cover the lesions to some degree, but removal of them is often more desirable. A single vein may feed a whole nest of other veins so that entry of one vein may provide access to the whole for injection purposes. An insulin syringe with 26-gauge needle is used. Sodium morrhuate is the only available injection material that is useful. Other agents are forthcoming pending regulatory approval. The risk of injection therapy is the extravasation of the material into the dermis at the time of injection or the subsequent leakage of the material from the puncture site with the same effect of producing sclerosis of the dermis with skin slough. This complication should be carefully explained to the patient because it may be unavoidable with this form of therapy. Laser therapy is used by some to avoid complications of skin slough which often accompany injection therapy, but the laser energy will produce unavoidable scar tattoo of the skin where it is applied. The procedure is performed with the patient lying on the procedure table. Several operating sessions may be required to eradicate all or most of the lesions. The length of each session is determined by the endurance of patient or operator. The site of injection is prepared with alcohol swab. The needle is introduced through the dermis until the tiny vein is punctured. This must be seen as it is not possible to withdraw blood conveniently through an insulin syringe. A small amount of sclerosing solution is injected and intravascular location is confirmed by observing the vein fill with colorless solution. More of the solution is injected while massaging the lesion to direct the solution to as much of the lesion as possible. After the needle is withdrawn, pressure is applied. The patient is left lying down for 20–30 minutes to assure hemostasis after the procedure. Subsequent injection sessions are scheduled at 3–6 weeks depending on the rate at which dermal inflammation resolves.

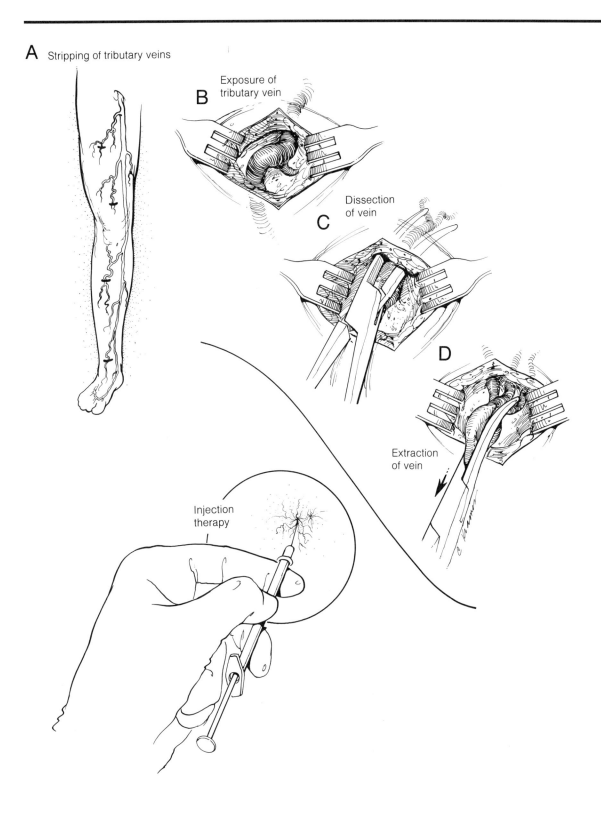

A Stripping of tributary veins

B Exposure of tributary vein

C Dissection of vein

D Extraction of vein

Injection therapy

Subfascial Ligation of Perforating Veins

Fig 35–3. Incompetence of the valves in the perforating veins that communicate the deep and superficial venous systems in the leg are usually responsible for leg edema, stasis dermatitis, and recurrent ulceration of the skin near the ankle. Division of the perforating veins relieves the venous hypertension to the skin and may allow chronic stasis ulcers to heal.

A. The classic approach for ligation of perforating veins in the subfascial plane was described by Linton. A medially placed incision in the leg below the knee somewhat posterior to the tibia and extending to the ankle was utilized. The incision usually passes right through chronically ulcerated skin.

B. A more favorable approach is that of Dodd. A long incision is made in the posterior calf midline of the skin of the leg below the knee. Over the area occupied by the Achilles tendon, the incision deviates medially so that healing will not create adhesion to the tendon. This approach has the advantage of being made posteriorly through the best skin in venous stasis syndrome. Incision of the ulcer is avoided. All of the perforating veins can be easily interrupted.

C. The incision is made through skin, subcutaneous tissue, and fascia with care taken not to raise a flap between skin and fascia. Fascial flaps are elevated. Perforating veins are identified as they rise from the deep venous circulation through the muscle of the leg. The perforating veins are ligated with hemoclips and divided.

D. A finger is inserted beneath the fascial flaps to disrupt any remaining perforating veins that have not been identified and divided. The dissection must be thorough and extend all the way around the leg to the tibia anteriorly on both medial and lateral aspects of the leg. The lesser saphenous vein may be ligated in the popliteal fossa. Closure of fascia and skin are routine. Skin grafts may be required for ulcerated skin.

Venous Valve Transposition

Operations on venous valves are in evolution. Operative technique is by no means standardized. Indications for these procedures are not completely established. Which operations to perform and long-term results are in question. One promising operation is illustrated here.

A. A longitudinal incision is made in the upper arm 4 cm below the axilla to expose the brachial vein. A 2-cm segment of vein that contains a valve is excised.

B. A medial approach to the popliteal vein is utilized. The incision extends across the knee exactly as for exposure of the popliteal artery. Heparin is administered intravenously to achieve systemic anticoagulation. A segment of the popliteal vein is excised. The brachial vein containing a competent valve is interposed between the ends of the popliteal vein. Meticulous end-to-end anastomosis is constructed using 6/0 or 7/0 polypropylene. An intermittent pneumatic compression device is used to augment venous flow after operation.

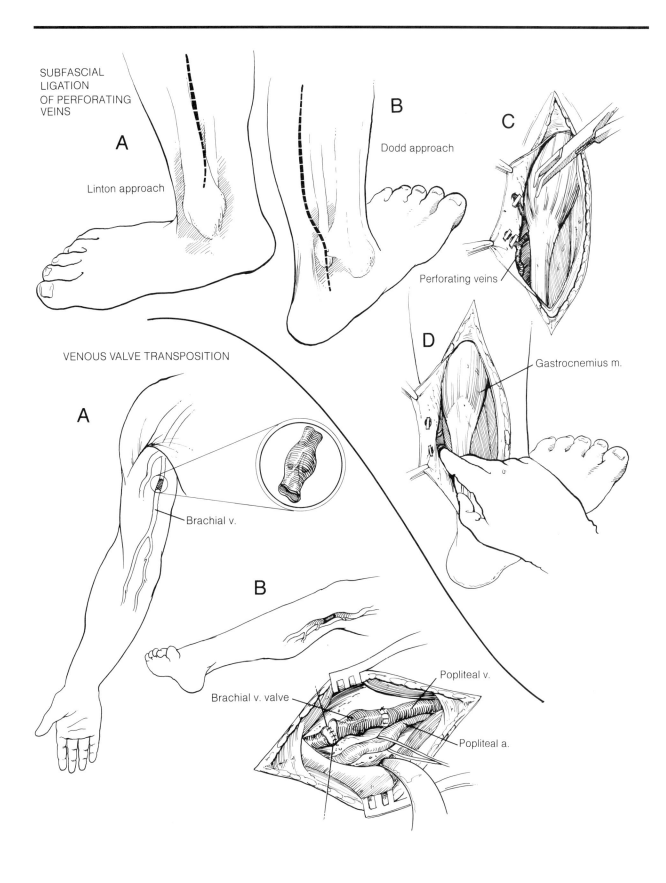

SUBFASCIAL
LIGATION
OF PERFORATING
VEINS

A

Linton approach

B

Dodd approach

C

Perforating veins

D

Gastrocnemius m.

VENOUS VALVE TRANSPOSITION

A

Brachial v.

B

Brachial v. valve

Popliteal v.

Popliteal a.

36

Inferior Vena Cava Interruption

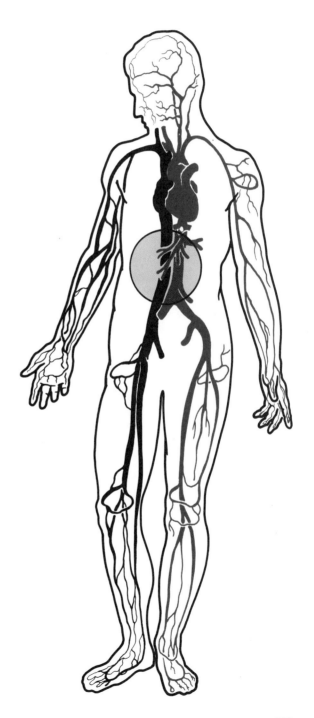

Fig 36–1. Interruption of the inferior vena cava is occasionally required for recurrent pulmonary embolism. Adequate anticoagulation with heparin will usually stop pulmonary embolism, prevent propagation of thrombus, and promote resolution of thrombus. Continuous intravenous infusion of heparin with activated clotting time approximately two times control level is the desired endpoint. Should pulmonary embolism occur on this medical regimen, operative intervention is indicated for patients having thrombosis in the veins of the legs or pelvis.

Interruption of the inferior vena cava by catheter technique under fluoroscopic control is the most popular technique. The catheter is inserted by cutdown over the right internal jugular vein. New catheter techniques which introduce a large sheath in the internal jugular or femoral vein may allow placement of these devices without cutdown.

A.   The sternal and clavicular heads of the sternocleido-mastoid muscle are separated exposing the internal jugular vein. The anterior surface of the vein is mobilized to free up enough tissue to allow placement of vascular occlusion clamps.

B.   A purse-string stitch is placed in the adventitia of the vein using 3/0 polypropylene suture. A tourniquet is attached. The jugular vein is controlled with angled peripheral vascular clamps (DeBakey) to isolate the area containing the purse-string. An incision is made within the purse-string.

C.   The capsule of the catheter occlusion device is inserted into the jugular vein. The vascular clamp located inferiorly is released to allow passage of the catheter device into the superior vena cava while controlling blood loss from the vein by the tourniquet on the purse-string stitch. Presently, the Greenfield catheter occlusion device is favored because of the reliability and ease of placement of the device in the inferior vena cava and because this device provides sufficient obstruction to prevent embolism without totally occluding the cava. During catheter insertion, it is important to keep the capsule flush line well irrigated with saline solution containing heparin in order to prevent thrombus formation on the filter device which may prevent it from opening properly to engage the wall of the inferior vena cava.

D.   Under fluoroscopic control, the catheter is passed through the superior vena cava and right atrium into the inferior vena cava and located just below the junction of the renal veins. Radiologic techniques which aid accurate placement of the capsule containing the occlusion device include: (1) inferior vena cavography at the time of pulmonary angiography with placement of the infusion to reflux contrast media to the renal veins; (2) placement of radiopaque markers on the skin to localize the renal vein junction and the caval bifurcation; (3) comparison of the cavagram to the skeletal structures to locate the renal vein junction relative to the vertebrae; and (4) determine the diameter of the cava from the cavagram for the proper size and selection of occlusion device.

E.   The occlusion device is pushed out of the capsule only part way at first so as to be sure that the device will release at the proper location. The capsule is pulled back while holding the internal catheter in place.

F.   The capsule is withdrawn leaving the occlusion device lodged against the walls of the inferior vena cava below the renal veins. The guide wire is left in the filter while withdrawing the capsule and until the device opens. Should the filter fail to open properly, the capsule with guide wire can be used to push the device into the femoral vein where it may be retrieved.

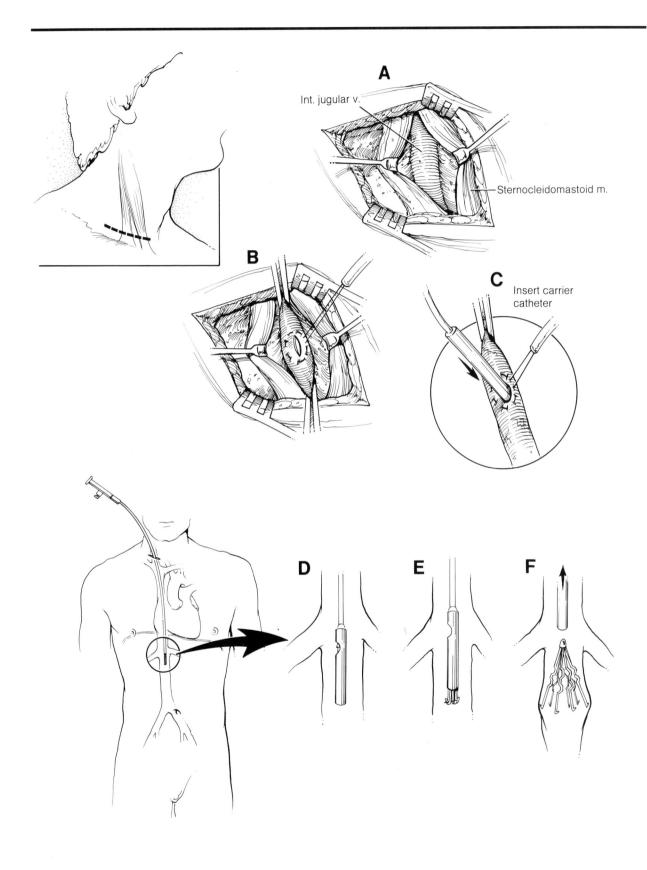

A

Int. jugular v.

Sternocleidomastoid m.

B

C

Insert carrier catheter

D

E

F

Fig 36–2. Operative interruption of the inferior vena cava is performed through a transverse incision on the right side of the abdomen opposite the umbilicus extending into the right flank.

A. The dissection is in the retroperitoneal space. The muscles of the abdominal wall are split and retracted, dividing muscle only as necessary to obtain required exposure. The peritoneum is left intact and a space developed between the peritoneum and the muscles of the abdominal wall. The cava is approached anterior to the psoas muscle. The ureter is retracted anteriorly with the peritoneal contents. The inferior vena cava is freed up enough to identify the left renal vein. It is controlled by passing a clamp around it at that point.

B. A small catheter is drawn around the cava just below the left renal vein. A plication clip is attached to the catheter by threading the catheter over one end of the device. The catheter is withdrawn from the cava, thereby guiding the plication clip around the inferior vena cava.

C. The plication clip is closed around the cava and the closure secured. The inferior vena cava is partially occluded by this technique.

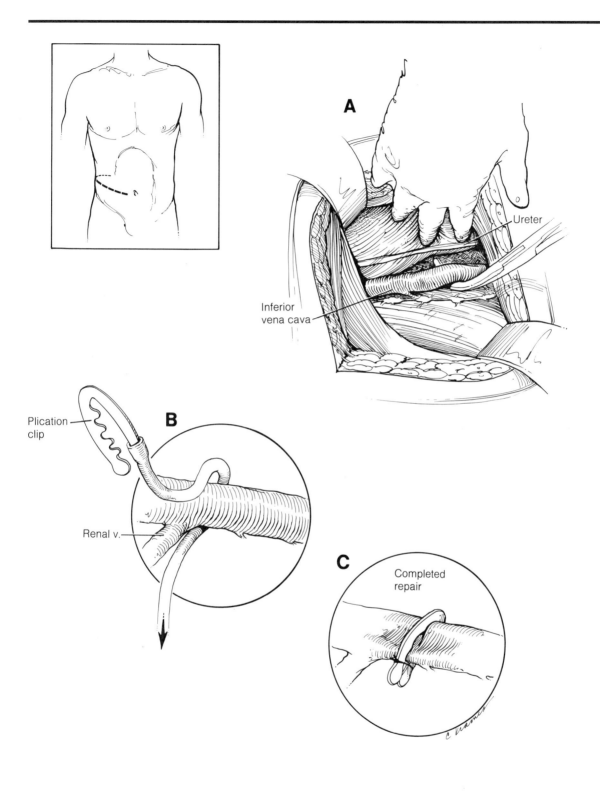

A

Ureter

Inferior vena cava

B

Plication clip

Renal v.

C

Completed repair

Index

Clamps, 4, 5
Claudication
	of calf, caused by popliteal artery entrapment, 200–203
	femoro-popliteal artery bypass for, 148–162
Coarctation, of proximal abdominal aorta, 120
Common hepatic artery aneurysm, 268, 269
Compartments, of leg
	anatomy, 284, 285
	lateral fasciotomy, 288, 289
	limited anterior fasciotomy, 286–287
	posterior fasciotomy, 288, 289
Composite graft procedures
	femoral artery and saphenous vein bypass graft, 188–189
	for insufficient saphenous vein, 184–187
	spiral saphenous vein graft construction, 316, 317
Control of blood vessels, 8–9 see also specific operative procedure
Cooley pediatric anastomosis clamp, 4, 6
Counter traction, 8, 9

D

Dacron graft, 98
DeBakey clamps, 4, 5
DeBakey forceps, 8, 9
Decompression, of neurovascular bundle, 312, 313
Derra anastomosis clamp, 4
Diethrich microcoronary bulldog clamp, 6
Dodd approach to subfascial ligation of perforating veins, 327
Doppler ultrasound blood flow velocity monitoring
	of bypass graft, 160, 178
	of external carotid endarterectomy, 20
	of inferior mesenteric artery, 208
	of renal artery, 96
Duodenum
	fistula formation, 102
	separation from false aneurysm and fistula, 142, 143

E

Electroencephalogram, intraoperative, 14
Embolectomy
	aortic bifurcation, 274–277
	arterial, 273
	brachial-radial-ulnar arterial, 280–381
	femoro-popliteal arterial, 278–279
	renal artery, 252, 253
Embolectomy catheter, 134
Embolus
	sites, 274, 275
	of superior mesenteric artery, 256
Endarterectomy
	aorto-iliac, 105–109
	aorto-renal, 248–249
	blind, 106, 108
	carotid, 13–17
		of aortic origin, 48–49
		with carotid-subclavian bypass, 42–43
		external, 19–22

in subclavian artery-external carotid artery bypass, 60, 61
innominate, of aortic origin, 48–49
instrumentation, 6, 7
of superficial femoral artery, 188
vertebral, 80, 81
Entrapment, of popliteal artery, 199–203
Exposure of blood vessels, 8, 9 see also specific operative procedure
Extensor digitorum longus muscle, anatomic relationships, 168, 169
Extra-anatomic bypass
	for aorto-enteric fistula reconstruction for intra-abdominal graft, 144–145
	ascending aorta-abdominal aorta, 120–123
	axillary-bilateral femoral artery, 118–119
	axillary-femoral artery, 114–115
	femoral-femoral artery, 112–113
	operative procedure, 111–123
Extracranial cerebral vascular procedures
	for aortic arch occlusive disease, 47–69
		endarterectomy of aortic origin of innominate or carotid artery, 48–49
	for carotid aneurysm, 29–36
	carotid artery bypass, 38–45
	for carotid body tumor, 71–76
	carotid endarterectomy, 13–17
	for carotid fibrodysplasia, 23–28
	carotid-subclavian bypass, 37–45
	external carotid endarterectomy, 19–21
	vertebral artery revascularization, 77–81

F

False aneurysm
	aortoenteric fistula and, 142
	femoral anastomotic, 136–137
	prevention of, 102, 210
Fasciotomy
	forearm, 290–291
	of lateral compartment, 288, 289
	limited, of anterior compartment, 286–287
	operative procedure, 283–291
	of posterior compartment, 288, 289
Femoral artery
	bifurcation, embolectomy, 278–279
	bypass
		using anterior tibial artery, 168–171
		using common femoral artery, 112–113
		using distal arteries, 126, 163–189
		using dorsalis pedis artery, 176–179
		using peroneal artery, 172–175
		using popliteal and posterior tibial artery, sequentially, 180–183
		using popliteal artery, 147–162
		using posterior tibial artery, 164–167
	common
		aorto-enteric fistula reconstruction for graft, 144–145
		control of, 96, 97
	composite saphenous vein bypass graft, 188–189
	false aneurysm at graft anastomosis, repair of, 136–137